John Geyman's justifi⟨ form' role of President Trump and his ᴋᴇᴘᴜᴜᴌ... ing. TrumpCare is what the ACA has become. This book explains why that is so regrettable.

—Theodore Marmor, Ph.D., professor emeritus of public policy and management at Yale University, author of *The Politics of Medicare* (2013), and member of the National Academy of Medicine

ObamaCare, TrumpCare. When are we going to get America-Care? We are running out of time and options. Working Americans and their families deserve better. Dr. Geyman shows us how we can all have accessible, high quality and affordable health care insurance. American families deserve better than our expensive and unfair patchwork of unpredictable plans and benefits. Meanwhile American businesses are saddled with unnecessary health care expenses making it hard to be competitive. Read this book from a wise family doctor to find out how we can create a better future for our loved ones, our economy and our country.

—Charles North, M.D., MS, Indian Health Service Chief Medical Officer, retired Captain USPHS, professor of family and community medicine, University of New Mexico

For many years Dr. John Geyman has been one of the sharpest observers and most convincing critics of American health care. *TrumpCare* is no exception. I recommend this excellent book to the lay public and policy makers alike. It makes crystal clear the health care collapse to which we are headed and how to avert it.

—Larry R. Churchill, professor of medical ethics emeritus, Vanderbilt University Medical Center

Amazingly prolific and indefatigably activist on behalf of health care as a human right, John Geyman has done it again. In *TrumpCare*, he uses his all-points knowledge of the American health care dilemma to out the waste, expense, profiteering, loss of coverage, and hypocrisy that is TrumpCare. He makes a powerful case that single-payer Medicare for All is the clear road out of the snake oil swamp concocted by the Charlatan-in-Chief.

—Fitzhugh Mullan, M.D., professor of health policy and management, and pediatrics at The George Washington University, and Board Chair of the Beyond Flexner Alliance

Despite repeated failures by the Republican-controlled Congress to repeal the Affordable Care Act outright, the war of attrition against Democratic attempts to expand healthcare coverage to more Americans continues, often under the radar and behind the scenes, or camouflaged by the ongoing circus in the nation's capitol. Dr. John Geyman's latest book, *TrumpCare*, brings them all out into the light. In it, he explores how TrumpCare has happened, what exactly it is, and why it will fail. He then offers an analysis of the healthcare policy choices that now face the American people and our political leaders, and persuasively explains why there is really only one viable option. At the end of the book, he quotes Richard Painter, a long time Republican and professor of law who recently switched parties to run for the US Senate: "This isn't about being a Democrat. I am an American before party... I'm not interested in party loyalty. I'm interested in policy, in issues, and in the right thing to do." I couldn't agree more.

—Phillip Caper, M.D., internist with long experience in health policy since the 1970s, and past chairman of the National Council on Health Planning and Development

In *TrumpCare*, John P. Geyman convincingly shows how our health care system, already failing during the Obama years, has deteriorated even further because of actions taken by the early Trump administration. He also argues cogently for the creation of a single-payer health care system to address our most pressing needs. This is a thoughtful and compelling analysis that merits attention by patients, providers, and payers of health care.

—Kenneth Ludmerer, M.D., professor of medicine and the history of medicine at Washington University in St. Louis, and past president of the American Association for the History of Medicine

John Geyman is relentless. He insists on an American healthcare system that reflects reliability, integrity, and competence, all of which are lacking in our current system and in our current White House leadership. Anyone who insists that TrumpCare is the greatest advance in medicine since ObamaCare should spend a few sobering moments with Dr. Geyman's latest book. No one does better at describing the vacuum at the head of our country. And no one does better at illuminating the way to better care for more people for less money.

—Samuel Metz, M.D., adjunct associate professor of anesthesiology,
Oregon Health and Science University, Portland, OR

Our overpriced but underperforming health care system is being made worse under Trump policies. It is extremely urgent that we change direction. John Geyman explains what has gone wrong and what we can do about it so that absolutely everyone finally can have affordable, high quality health care.

—Don McCanne, M.D., family physician, senior health policy fellow
and past president of Physicians for a National Health Program (PNHP)

I found this book excellent and plan to keep it close at hand for reference. Perhaps as single-payer comes more into general acceptance we as doctors can focus more on details not in legislation, particularly the need for a national electronic medical records system and a national professional consensus on appropriate care.

—Jim Burdick, M.D., professor of surgery at
Johns Hopkins University School of Medicine

Winston Churchill supposedly said, "You can always count on the Americans to do the right thing, after they have exhausted all other possibilities." As Dr. Geyman shows in detail, now that TrumpCare has replaced ObamaCare, we are rapidly exhausting all other possibilities. One hopes that the right thing, which Dr. Geyman also describes, will now not be long in coming.

—Howard Brody, M.D., Ph.D, Director of the Institute for Medical
Humanities, University of Texas Medical Branch, Galveston, TX

All my career, policy wonks have tinkered with ways to improve market-based healthcare. This has brought us the highest costs in the world, with access and quality inferior to those in most advanced countries. The Trump administration is racing to make things worse, while claiming the opposite. Dr. Geyman demonstrates, with ample evidence, why the proposed changes will reduce access and quality, while driving patient costs (and corporate profits) into the ionosphere. His lucid explanations, recommendations, and real facts should be required reading for policymakers and anyone concerned about their health care.

—Richard A. Deyo M.D., MPH, professor emeritus, Department of Family Medicine, Department of Medicine, Oregon Health and Science University and author of *Watch Your Back! How the Back Pain Industry Is Costing Us More and Giving Us Less—and What You Can Do to Inform Yourself in Seeking Treatment*

The voice of Dr. John Geyman has been a consistent and clarion call for common sense in our solution to the crisis of our disintegrating and unsustainable healthcare system. In his latest work he has once again, thoroughly and dispassionately, laid out the most current facts in our national debate over healthcare reform. The battle lines have been drawn, Geyman argues, and the midterm elections of 2018 place us at a crucial crossroads, with a clear choice between TrumpCare, a continuing (and failed) "business model" of healthcare which serves the interests of the corporate few versus Medicare for All, an affordable and sustainable service model of healthcare which serves the common good, and provides universal coverage for all.

—Rick Flinders, M.D., family physician and former long-term educator at the Santa Rosa Family Medicine Residency, Sutter Santa Rosa Regional Hospital, Santa Rosa, CA

TRUMPCARE

Lies, Broken Promises, How It Is Failing, and What Should Be Done

John Geyman, M.D.

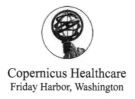

Copernicus Healthcare
Friday Harbor, Washington

TrumpCare
Lies, Broken Promises, How It Is Failing, and What Should Be Done

John Geyman, M.D.

Copernicus Healthcare
Friday Harbor, WA

First Edition

Book design, cover and illustrations by W. Bruce Conway
Cover image used under license from Shutterstock.com
Author photo by Anne Sheridan

softcover: ISBN 978-1-938218-18-7

Library of Congress Control Number: 2018954786

Copernicus Healthcare
34 Oak Hill Drive
Friday Harbor, WA 98250

www.copernicus-healthcare.org

DEDICATION

To the many millions of Americans struggling to gain access to necessary health care in our failing health care system designed to meet the needs of corporate interests, not those of us as patients. And to the hundreds of thousands of health care professionals trying to cope with a dysfunctional and bureaucratic system that takes their time away from serving patients. And to the growing army of citizen activists committed to health care reform. May this country find a way to finance health care that provides universal coverage for all Americans and returns medicine to its traditional ethic of service.

CONTENTS

HOW DID THIS HAPPEN?

WHAT IS TRUMP CARE?

HOW TRUMPCARE IS FAILING

WHAT NOW? JUST TWO OPTIONS AHEAD

Tables and Figures

Acknowledgements

As with my previous books, I am indebted to many for making this book possible. Thanks are especially due to many investigative journalists, health professionals, and others for their probing reports on our evolving, dysfunctional health care system. The work of many organizations has been useful in gathering evidence-based information on what is actually happening in U.S. health care, including the Kaiser Family Foundation, the Commonwealth Fund, the Center for National Health Program Studies, Public Citizen's Health Research Group, the Centers for Medicare and Medicaid Services, the U. S. Government Accountability Office, and the Congressional Budget Office.

W. Bruce Conway, my colleague at Copernicus Healthcare, has once again done a great job from start to finish of this project, including cover design, interior layout, and conversion to e-book format. Carolyn Acheson of Edmonds, Washington has again created a useful, reader-friendly index.

Most of all, I am grateful to my wife, Emily, for her helpful suggestions and encouragement throughout the process, including editing, proofing, and promotion of the book.

PREFACE

Since the Republican Congress has failed to repeal and replace the Affordable Care Act (ACA), or ObamaCare, over the last eight years, together with the first eighteen months of the Trump administration, there is widespread confusion and anger among the public as to what is really going on in health care. Most Americans are increasingly anxious about whether they can afford their own insurance and health care. Even those already covered by Medicare and Medicaid are worried about threatened cutbacks and increased costs as Congressional Republicans dedicate themselves to slashing "entitlement" funding to help pay down the $1.5 trillion deficit resulting from the 2017 passage of their tax bill.

In mid-October, 2017, President Trump issued an executive order intended to hasten the demise of ObamaCare. It called for government agencies to expand association health plans by allowing them to form groups across state lines, to expand the marketing of low-cost, barebones insurance for periods less than 12 months, and encourage wider use of health reimbursement accounts (HRAs) by employers for their employees. None of these directions will improve access to care or address systemic problems of high health care costs. We can expect that the federal government will increasingly shift the burden for health care to the states, likely through block grants, giving them more flexibility (and less accountability) for their own programs and "saving" the government money. As columnist David Leonhardt observed:

TrumpCare has begun, not through legislation but through executive action . . . In doing so, it has both the short-term goal (have the federal government do less to help vulnerable citizens) and a long-term goal (sabotage ObamaCare, so that Congress can more easily repeal the law). [1]

ObamaCare has been so undermined by past and ongoing actions of the Trump administration that we can no longer call the ACA ObamaCare. It is now TrumpCare, with Trump and Republicans in Congress owning it.

Lies have pervaded this unstable period under the false cloak of improving health care. As just one example, with the repeal of the ACA's individual mandate as part of the Republican tax cut bill in December, 2017, Trump bragged:

In this bill, not only do we have massive tax cuts and tax reform, we have essentially repealed ObamaCare, and we'll come up with something that is much better. ObamaCare has been repealed in this bill. [2]

As Trump claimed paternity for TrumpCare, the Congressional Budget Office projected that an additional 13 million people will lose their health insurance by 2026, by then not far from the 50 million uninsured before the ACA was enacted. Some insurers were exiting the market and premium increases were being announced by more than 50 percent in a number of states. It soon became clear that the tax cut bill would mainly benefit Wall Street, corporations and the wealthy, not the middle class or lower-income people. This will continue present trends, since health care stock prices have gone up almost four-fold since the ACA was enacted in 2010, compared to 116 percent increase in other sectors. [3]

Chaos reigns throughout our increasingly fragmented and dysfunctional health care system. Corporate mergers and profits are the order of the day, with the business "ethic" to make more money trumping the traditional service ethic of care. Health care is becoming less and less affordable or accessible, while Americans continue to lose free choice of physician, other providers, and hospitals. Family budgets are already strained to the limits as many patients forgo necessary care, have worse outcomes if and when they finally get care, and often have to choose between food and medications. The angry protests at town halls across the country last summer give us examples of the depth of this anger. Continuity of personal care over years has for many people become a thing of the past as fragmentation pervades the system.

Health care is a leading issue in the forthcoming 2018 midterm elections, and promises to be in the 2020 election cycle. This book undertakes four goals: (1) to describe what our increasingly dysfunctional health care system looks like after the ACA has been gutted by GOP sabotage; (2) to show how TrumpCare will fail patients, families, tax payers, and the nation; (3) to describe the increasing crisis in U. S. health care; and (4) to outline the only two future scenarios that could deal with this worsening situation, only one of which will work.

It is my hope that this book will help voters to better understand their options during the coming election cycles, as well as help candidates hoping to be elected to positions where they can make a difference.

—John Geyman, M.D.
Friday Harbor, WA
August, 2018

References

1. Leonhardt, D. How to fight the new TrumpCare. *New York Times*, October 15, 2017.
2. Trump, D. J. as quoted by Cunningham, P W. A eulogy for the individual mandate. *The Washington Post*, December 21, 2017.
3. Phelan, M. *Social Security Works*, August 5, 2017.

How Did This Happen?

CHAPTER 1

HISTORICAL PERSPECTIVE

*If you can't take care of your sick in the country, forget it,
it's all over. I mean, it's no good. So I'm very liberal when it
comes to healthcare. I believe in universal healthcare. I believe
in whatever it takes to make people well and better.*

—Donald Trump, in a 1999 interview with Larry King Live[1]

Here is Trump in the above quote almost 20 years ago, as a multimillionaire or billionaire, posturing as a pseudo populist. He was seeming to support universal health care, but lying through his teeth as he has done regularly since running for president and in his first presidential year. With all that supposed dedication to universal health care, why have we seen no progress toward health care reform in Trump's first year as president? As we all know so well, he has very little knowledge about policy in any area, changes his mind via tweets on a frequent, even daily basis, and appears to have no historical knowledge or principles of his own. His 1999 statement was as uninformed and incoherent as we see every day today on a wide range of subjects. Now he is fighting against any effort to broaden health care in the public interest, quite the opposite of his earlier declaration. His administration, together with a Republican-controlled Congress, is committed to repealing the Affordable Care Act (ACA or ObamaCare) without any idea for a replacement plan.

This chapter has three goals: (1) to bring historical perspective to past efforts to reform U. S. health care and achieve universal health care in this country; (2) to discuss barriers to reform over those years; and (3) to consider what we can learn about these failed efforts over more than a century.

Historical Perspective

As candidate for president in 1912 with the Progressive Party, Theodore Roosevelt made National Health Insurance (NHI) a platform plank. The trend over the previous 30 years had been to establish similar programs in many European countries, usually as sickness insurance, with Germany the leader in 1883.

Although TR lost the 1912 election, a social insurance committee of the American Medical Association actually adopted this resolution in 1917:

> *The time is present when the profession should study earnestly to solve the questions of medical care that will arise under various forms of social insurance. Blind opposition, indignant repudiation, bitter denunciation of these laws is worse than useless; it leads nowhere and it leaves the profession in a position of helplessness as the rising tide of social development sweeps over it.* [2]

That resolution soon fell by the wayside as state chapters around the country denounced it, and the AMA has taken a reactionary position against national health insurance (NHI) ever since.

In the mid-1930s, President Franklin Delano Roosevelt considered including NHI in his New Deal agenda, but backed off because of strong opposition from the AMA. Since then, the only real NHI proposal was made by President Harry Truman in 1946, but it again failed as opponents lobbied a Republican controlled Congress and played to the public's neo-Cold War fears of "socialism." [3]

Later efforts to reform U. S. health care fell way short of NHI. In the early 1970s, President Nixon offered his own "Play or Pay" proposal as an alternative to Ted Kennedy's single-payer plan. It would have required employers to either offer acceptable coverage to their employees or pay a tax that would finance their coverage from an insurance pool that would also cover the unemployed. Besieged as he was with the Vietnam War and Watergate, Nixon's proposal went through several iterations in Congress only to fail to gain sufficient support for passage. [4]

The next major reform attempts in 1993-1994 included the Clinton Health Plan (CHP), a very complex proposal that combined employer mandates and spending controls. The Clinton plan attracted such intense controversy from most quarters that the 1,342 page bill never got out of committee to a vote in the House. It was strongly opposed by the insurance industry which fielded a national television campaign, "Harry and Louise", who sat around their kitchen table finding fault with the plan. Among several competing bills at the time, the single-payer plan proposed by Representative Jim McDermott (D-WA), the only one for NHI, had strong grassroots support, attracted the largest number of supporters in Congress, and was the only bill to pass out of committee. But it was soon lost in the shuffle and marginalized by the mainstream media as the war over the Clinton plan proceeded to its demise. [5]

Passage of the ACA was the signature domestic legislation of the Obama years. Democrats gave it strong support against an ongoing barrage of attacks by Republicans, who saw it as a "government takeover" when the opposite was true. Each health care industry profited immensely from the bill—insurers by gaining more enrollees and new streams of federal funding, hospitals by having more paying patients, and the drug industry by enlarging their markets and avoiding any price controls. Despite attacks from the GOP, some 24 million Americans gained access to care through becoming insured, especially through expansion of Medicaid in 31 states. Important patient protections were also included in the bill, such as banning insurers from denying coverage for pre-existing conditions and allowing parents to keep their children on their coverage until age 26.

Republicans in Congress continued to vow to repeal and replace the bill at the earliest possible time, but when their time came after the 2016 elections, they failed repeatedly in that quest despite controlling the White House and both chambers of Congress. Republican legislators were divided among themselves. The far right Freedom Caucus dug in over the need to cut Medicaid in the short and long term, further deregulate the insurance market to give consumers "more choice," shift control of health care back to the states through block grants, and defund Planned Parenthood. Moderate Republicans pushed back, fearing re-election losses if more than 22 million people were to lose insurance if the ACA was repealed. The GOP was in a further quandary by having no replacement plan of its own, the opposition to any of their proposals by corporate stakeholders in the ACA, and continued strong public support for the ACA with little support for GOP proposals. After their late January retreat at White Sulphur Springs, West Virginia, the Republican leadership said they would not pursue further health care legislation in an election year. [6]

Since the 2016 elections, Republicans have been steadfast in sabotaging the ACA in any number of ways, hoping that it will implode on its own. Their supposed tax cut plan did repeal the ACA's individual mandate, causing heartburn among insurers. Many administrative initiatives have also been taken, including decreasing funds promoting ACA enrollment, cutting enrollment periods from 90 to 45 days, discontinuing cost-sharing reduction (CSR) payments to insurers, and proposed new rules by The Centers for Medicare and Medicaid (CMS) that would allow states to set up their own plans without responding to the ACA's constraints.

The revolving door is still in effect. As one example, Seema Verma helped to implement Medicaid "reform" in Indiana while Michael Pence was Governor. She was picked by Trump to head the Centers for Medicare and Medicaid (CMS). In this capacity she presides over an almost $1 trillion annual budget, plans to further privatize and cut back Medicare and Medicaid, and give states more latitude to avoid the ACA's restraints on insurer practices.

At this writing (August 2018), the mid-term election campaigns are in high gear, with much of the electorate very concerned about the continued escalation of health care costs with no containment on the horizon. Health care is increasingly unaffordable for much of the population. With the health insurance market de-stabilized, many insurers are exiting the market, and a growing number of counties are bare without any insurer. Consolidation is gaining speed through mega mergers, with rising prices the result instead of lowering costs through "competition." As examples, the five largest health insurance companies almost quintupled since 2010. UnitedHealth, the nation's largest insurer by market share and the largest health care company in the world by revenue, is expanding its reach into ownership of medical practices, including surgery centers and urgent care clinics, and managing pharmacy benefits. [7]

The medical-industrial complex rolls on, with no significant reform yet to be seen in a paralyzed Congress, as corporate stakeholders continue to reap profits as a cash cow with no incentives to change, and as the Trump administration continues to sabotage the

ACA and pursues further deregulation.

The U. S. remains an outlier among all other advanced countries around the world in still not assuring universal access to health care. Western Europe and Scandinavian countries all have one or another system of universal health care, as do Canada, Taiwan, New Zealand, Australia, and other countries. This is especially ironic since health care was recognized as a human right way back in 1948, when the General Assembly of the United Nations adopted its Universal Declaration of Human Rights, which was later adopted as well by the World Health Organization in its Declaration of the Rights of Patients.

Barriers to Health Care Reform

We can better understand why these efforts to reform U. S. health care have failed over more than a century by considering some major contributing factors that have led to this result.

1. Myths and memes.

Many myths have evolved over the years and repeated so often as to become memes. Here are just three of the more important that still stand in the way of rational assessment of competing proposals.

The free market will fix our problems; competition works.

Many economists have held the belief over many years that health care markets work like other markets where competition can rein in prices and patients can shop for the best deal. In turn, most conservatives and those representing corporate stakeholders continue to promote this belief even though it has been fully discredited over the years for many reasons. Health care decision-making is not like shopping for the best deal on a new car. There is a knowledge gap between patients and health professionals, information is often unavailable, patients often don't know their needs, urgency of time is often a controlling factor as to who and where patients can access care, health insurers frequently restrict these choices, and consolidation of corporate providers invariably increases costs. Dr. Friedrich A Hayek, leading economist from the last century and professor of social and moral sciences at the University of Chicago, saw this coming as early as 1946:

> *Market capitalism will have the same inefficient, exploitive outcome as Soviet Communism if the ownership of resources becomes concentrated in the hands of fewer and fewer large corporations, and if economic business decisions come to be made by those relatively few individuals who own and/or operate large concentrated corporations.*[8]

The private sector is more efficient than the public sector.

Market enthusiasts have long promoted the idea that the private sector is more efficient and provides more value to consumers than the public sector. Traditional Medicare as enacted in 1965 for everyone age 65 and older gives us an excellent example that rebuts this myth. Over more than the last 50 years, it has been run with a low overhead of about 2.5 percent, and has proven to be a solid rock in a volatile health care marketplace. Compare this with private insurers that operate with administrative costs five times larger, restrict choice, cherry pick the market for favorable risk selection, impose higher deductibles and co-payments, dis-enroll sicker people, and withdraw from the market if it is not sufficiently profitable. [9]

People with insurance overuse health care services.

This assumption has underlain the conventional theory of health insurance based on the concept of "moral hazard", that holds that patients' behavior changes when they become insured, to the point that they abuse the system. The trend toward "consumer driven health care" (CDHC) in recent decades has been based on this premise, assuming that imprudent choices can be avoided when patients are more financially responsible for their decisions and have "more skin in the game." Policies have therefore been adopted throughout our system that require more cost-sharing by patients with the goal of reining in health care costs.

Though this myth persists today, experience over the last 30 years has shown the failure of this approach to contain health care costs. Instead, more cost-sharing with patients leads many to forgo or delay necessary care, resulting in higher costs down the road and worse outcomes. We have also yet to admit that the purpose of higher deductibles is not to help patients but to decrease spending by insurers, employers, and government plans. [10]

2.   Health care by corporations

Corporatization and growth of for-profit health care has been the dominant trend in the U. S. over the last four decades. Corporate hospital chains were established within a few years after the enactment of Medicare and Medicaid in 1965. As the profits of investor-owned facilities and services grew rapidly, Wall Street became closely involved. Between 1965 and 1990, their corporate profits grew by more than 100 times, a pace almost 20 times greater than profits for all U. S. corporations. [11]

As Paul Starr, professor of sociology and public affairs at Princeton University, noted as early as 1982:

The rise of a corporate ethos in medical care is already one of the most significant consequences of the changing structure of medical care. It permeates voluntary hospitals, government agencies, and academic thought as well as profit-making medical care organizations. Those who talked about "health care planning" in the 1970s now talk about "health care marketing." Everywhere one sees the growth of a kind of marketing mentality in health care. And, indeed, business school graduates are displacing graduates of public health schools, hospital administrators, and even doctors in the top echelons of medical care organizations. The organizational culture of medicine used to be dominated by the ideals of professionalism and voluntarism, which softened the underlying acquisitive activity. The restraint exercised by those ideals grew weaker. The "health center" of one era is the "profit center" of the next.[12]

Some readers may be surprised how extensive for-profit ownership had become by 2016 across our health care system: specialty hospitals (37 percent), hospice (63 percent), nursing homes (65 percent), home care (76 percent), dialysis (90 percent), SurgiCenters (95 percent), and free-standing laboratory and imaging centers (100 percent). [13]

3. *Medical-industrial complex, with corporate economic and political power allied with Wall Street.*

In 1980, the late Dr. Arnold Relman, internist and former editor of *The New England Journal of Medicine*, coined the term "medical-industrial complex." He did so in describing the emergence of a new for-profit health care industry ranging from proprietary hospitals and nursing homes to diagnostic services, medical devices, hemodialysis, and the pharmaceutical and insurance industries. He gave us this warning 38 years ago:

> *This new "medical-industrial complex" may be more efficient than its not-for-profit competition, but it creates the problems of overuse and fragmentation of services, over emphasis on technology, and "cream skimming," and it may also exercise undue influence on national health policy. Closer attention from the public and the profession, and careful study are necessary to ensure that the "medical-industrial complex" puts the interests of the public before those of its stockholders.* [14]

4. Health care as a commodity, not a service

A sea change has occurred over the last four decades in this country which has taken the medical profession and health care from a cottage industry to a complex industry largely driven by business goals of profitability and financial bottom lines that are increasingly driven by the needs of investors. Health care has been reduced to a commodity for sale on an open market that is mostly controlled by ever-larger corporations. Almost two-thirds of physicians today are employees of these organizations, especially hospital systems with their affiliated ambulatory care facilities. As employees, they are subject to their employers' drive to increase their revenues.

5. Health care as large part of the economy

The health care industry has become a large part of the U.S. economy. More than one-third of the nation's job growth since the recession hit in late 2007 has been in the health sector, the single biggest sector for job growth. As the system has become more complex and fragmented, it has become administratively top-heavy, with 16 other workers for every physician. One half of these are in administrative and other non-clinical roles, especially involving data entry and other aspects related to billing and reimbursement. [15]

Privatization of public programs, such as Medicare and Medicaid, is another feature of this new environment. We have evolved a system of corporate welfare for the insurance, hospital, pharmaceutical and other industries that feeds on public programs at taxpayer expense. Two-thirds of U. S. health care costs are now paid for by the government—with our taxes. [16]

Takeaway Lessons from Failed Health Care Reform

What can we learn from the battles over health care reform, particularly since the Clinton effort in the 1990s and the ACA in 2008-2010? There are definite parallels with today's battles and here are eight obvious takeaway lessons that we need to learn if we are to be successful in future reform efforts.

1. *Previous reform attempts have been hijacked by corporate stakeholders*

Taking the ACA as an example, the interests of private insurers, hospitals, drug and medical device industries, organized medicine, and other stakeholders in our market-based system took precedence over the needs of patients for broad access to affordable, quality health care. The political process that led up to passage of the ACA involving the corporate alliance of the Big Four—the insurance industry, PhRMA, the hospital industry, and organized medicine—was described in my 2010 book, *Hijacked: The Road to Single Payer in the Aftermath of Stolen Health Care Reform*. [17] Bob Herbert, well-known Op-Ed columnist for the *New York Times*, was spot on with this observation:

The drug companies, the insurance industry and the rest of
the corporate high-rollers have their tentacles all over this so-
called reform effort, squeezing it for all its worth. Meanwhile,
the public—struggling with the worst economic downturn since
the 1930s—is looking on with great anxiety and confusion. If the
drug companies and the insurance industry are smiling, it can
only mean that the public interest is being left behind. [18]

Lobbying and influence peddling in the Beltway was rampant
as the ACA was being framed and crafted. Based on ideology
and political forces, there was never any likelihood that the new
marketplace could bring the needed reforms. It was a given that what
was spent on lobbying would bring far more revenue than its costs.
Robert Field, professor of law and of health policy and management
at Drexel University, observed:

The ACA set the stage for a financial boon for the health
care industry in numerous ways. It enables millions of new cus-
tomers to purchase individual policies. It permits Medicaid pro-
grams in many states to retain more managed care companies
to administer benefits.

It helps hospitals and many physicians to realize increased
revenues by giving more of their patients access to the finan-
cial resources needed to pay for care. And, over time, countless
other businesses will emerge and thrive under the ACA's gov-
ernment-created structure as the ingenuity of the private sector
finds ways to thrive off its new public base. [19]

2. You can't contain costs by permitting for-profit health care industries to pursue their business ethic in a deregulated market.

As one could have expected from long experience in this country, markets have completely failed to rein in prices and costs of

health care. Quite the opposite as they have continued to escalate for hospitals, physicians, drug and medical device manufacturers and other parts of our system. One venture capitalist promoting investment opportunities for private exchanges under the ACA saw the likelihood to "turn chaos into gold." [20] That is exactly what happened as health care stocks soared by almost 40 percent in 2013, the highest of any sector in the S & P 500. [21]

3. *You can't reform the delivery system without reforming the financing system.*

The U. S. keeps missing the boat in trying to contain health care costs within a largely for-profit multi-payer financing system. Our attempts to reform the delivery system so as to cover more people at more affordable costs proves to be futile every time it is tried. In the aftermath of the ACA's enactment eight years ago, the private health insurance industry has become even more complex and intrusive as it continues to profit from new subsidized markets. Insurers keep trying to avoid sicker, costlier patients and gaming the system to maximize their profits and keep their shareholders happy.

In true health care reform, our goal should be to provide universal access for our entire population to affordable, quality care without discrimination against the sick, those with pre-existing conditions, the poor, or the unemployed. Dr. Samuel Metz, adjunct associate professor of anesthesiology at Oregon Health and Science University in Portland, offers these three rules to achieve financing reform, all based on the solid experience over many years in advanced countries around the world that have transparent, publicly accountable, not-for-profit financing systems:

1. If you want comprehensive care for more people for less money, reform the financing system.

*2. If you want a dramatic reduction in costs without compro-
mising quality, reform the delivery system.*

3. If you want Rule # 2 to work, you must first apply Rule # 1.[22]

**4. In order to achieve the most efficient health insurance
coverage, we need to have the largest possible risk pool.**

The larger and more diverse the risk pool, the more effective
insurance can be in having healthier people share the costs of sicker people and keeping costs down. We know that 20 percent of the
population accounts for 80 percent of all health care spending, while
5 percent of the population uses almost one-half of total spending.
[23] As long as we have a large private insurance industry with some
1,300 insurers trying to avoid sicker patients, with millions of younger, healthier people choosing to be uninsured, we will have segmented risk pools that prevent efficiencies of a large risk pool. As other
advanced countries have found years ago, sharing risk across their
whole populations is the only way to provide universal coverage at
affordable costs to patients, families, and taxpayers.

**5. We can no longer afford to keep bailing out a failed private
health insurance industry.**

The multi-payer health insurance industry stands in the way of
universal coverage, is obsolete, and provides insufficient value to be
continuously bailed out by government and taxpayers. The industry
has had a long run since the 1960s, when it adopted medical underwriting practices to avoid sicker people with the goal of increased
profits. Today it is antithetical to reform as it games a subsidized
financing system for higher revenues for its CEOs and shareholders
on the backs of patients and taxpayers.

The government has been more than friendly to the industry
for many years through such perks as long-standing tax exemp-

tions for employer-sponsored insurance and overpayments to Medicare Advantage plans. The ACA increased these subsidies in more ways, including passing along cost-sharing reduction (CSR) payments, new "risk corridor" payments to protect insurers from losses, and expansion of private Medicare and Medicaid plans. Under the ACA, insurers have still found ways to game the system for higher profits by such means as high cost sharing, inadequate provider networks, denial of services, restrictive drug formularies, manipulation of risk scores to get higher Medicare payments, marketing short-term plans lasting less than one year as a way to avoid the ACA's requirements, and deceptive marketing practices. Even while continuing to receive large subsidies from the government, the industry consumes 15 to 20 percent of the health care dollar in bureaucracy, administrative overhead, and profits as it retains a top position on Wall Street's S & P 500.

The cost of private health insurance has become prohibitive for much of the population, even as its coverage becomes skinnier all the time. The costs of insurance and health care now account for almost one-half of average household income for families of four. Insurers have factored in the loss of CSR subsidies, with large premium increases for 2018—116 percent in Arizona and more than 50 percent in other states. Insurers are pushing to offer barebones policies, and we have an epidemic of *underinsurance*. Aetna, the nation's third largest insurer, scaled back its coverage even after its second-quarter 2017 revenue jumped by 52 percent. [24] Mark Bertolini, Aetna's CEO, recently acknowledged that the ACA's exchanges are in a "death spiral." [25] More insurers are leaving markets, with about one-half of U. S. counties having only one insurer this year, while we can expect to see a growing number of bare counties without any insurers. Wendell Potter, former industry insider, sums up the future of the industry this way:

Folks, we are guilty of magical thinking. We've fallen for insurers' deception and misdirection, hook, line, and sinker. And many of us can't be persuaded that we are being duped. Meanwhile, the shareholders of the big for-profits are laughing all the way to the bank. Every single day. [26]

6. Access to buying health insurance is not coverage if you can't afford it.

After the continued failures of the Republican-controlled Congress to repeal and replace the ACA, together with their inability to come up with any coherent replacement plan, the GOP has brought forward the vague and deceptive concept that "everyone should have the opportunity to buy health insurance if they so choose." This would be a fraudulent policy of "universal access," without any regard to affordability or quality of that coverage. During his nomination hearing before the Senate, Dr. Tom Price said:

I believe that every single American has access to the highest quality care and coverage that is possible. [27]

This flawed concept is ludicrous and will go nowhere, as it completely fails to recognize that the cost of insurance and care for a typical family of four with employer-sponsored insurance is now about $28,000 a year (almost one-half of median household income). Universal access mean nothing if people cannot afford insurance and care. As a result, many millions of people forgo or delay necessary care because of costs, and end up with worse outcomes if and when they finally do get care.

7. We *need a larger, not smaller, role of government to reform health care.*

The obvious failure of market-based policies and deregulation to contain health care costs and make them affordable for Americans over these many years calls for a larger role of government if we are ever to achieve real universal access to health care in this country. It is beyond time to acknowledge that the neoconservative policies of past, recent, and current administrations have not worked. Corporate interests in the medical-industrial complex stand in the way of universal access as they continue on their profit-taking binge with little public accountability. Today's market-based system leaves an ever-larger part of the population without needed care, and is unsustainable. We have yet to accept the necessity of government to assure that the public interest is being met. As Jacob Hacker, PhD, professor of political science at Yale University, recently observed:

> *The difference between the United States and other countries isn't the role of insurance; it's the role of government. More specifically, it's the way in which those who benefit from America's dysfunctional market have mobilized to use government to protect their earnings and profits . . . But in every other rich country, the government not only provides coverage to all citizens; it also provides strong counter pressure to those who seek to use their inherent market power to raise prices or deliver lucrative but unnecessary services . . .* [28]

8. *Failed health care reform exposes our loss of the democratic process.*

The Trump administration is clearly bent on dismantling our democratic institutions, battling against the norms of judicial process, and fighting against the free press in an increasingly dictatorial approach to governance. As David Frum has said in his 2018 book, *Trumpocracy: The Corruption of the American Republic*:

> *As President Trump is cruel, vengeful, egoistic, ignorant, lazy, avaricious and treacherous, so we must be kind, forgiving, responsible, informed, hardworking, generous, and patriotic. As Trump's enablers are careless, cynical, shortsighted, morally obtuse, and rancorous, so Trump's opponents must be thoughtful, idealistic, wise, morally sensitive, and conciliatory.* [29]

Noam Chomsky, Ph.D., professor emeritus of linguistics and philosophy at the Massachusetts Institute of Technology and author of the 2016 book, *Who Rules the World?*, brings this perspective to our circumstances and political challenges today:

> *Beginning in the 1970s, partly because of the economic crisis that erupted in the early years of that decade and the decline in the rate of profit, but also partly because of the view that democracy had become too widespread, an enormous, concentrated, coordinated business offensive was begun to try to beat back the egalitarian efforts of the post-war era,which only intensified as time went on. The economy itself shifted to financialization. Financial institutions expanded enormously. By 2007 right before the crash for which they had considerable responsibility, financial institutions accounted for a stunning 40 percent of corporate profit. A vicious cycle between concentrated capital and politics accelerated, while increasingly wealth concentrated in the financial sector. Politicians, faced with the rising cost of campaigns, were driven ever deeper into the pockets of wealthy backers. And politicians rewarded them by pushing policies favorable to Wall Street and other powerful business interests. Throughout this period, we have a renewed*

form of class warfare directed by the business class against the working people and the poor, along with a conscious attempt to roll back the gains of previous decades. [30]

Professor Chomsky's astute observation leads us directly into the next chapter, where we will consider how health policy in this country is bought and sold by the highest bidders.

References:

1. Rechtoris, M. 8 Donald Trump quotes on healthcare—'Repeal it, replace it, get something great! *Becker's Hospital Review*, August 16, 2016.

2. Burrow, JG. AMA: *Voice of American Medicine*. Baltimore. *Johns Hopkins Press*, 1963:144.

3. Thai, KV, Qiao, Y, McManus, SM. National health care reform failure: The political economy perspective. *J Health Hum Serv Adm*. Fall 1998: 21 (2): 236-259.

4. Iglehart, JK. Compromise seems unlikely on three major insurance plans. *National Journal Reports*. May 11, 1974; 6: 700-707.

5. Brundin, J. How the U. S. press covers the Canadian health care system. *Int J Health Serv* 1993; 23(2): 275-277.

6. Everett, B. Republicans give up on Obamacare repeal. *Politico,* February 1, 2018.

7. Terhune, C. Health companies race to catch UnitedHealth as Amazon laces up. *Kaiser Health News*, November 3, 2017.

8. Hayek, FA. The use of knowledge in society. *Am Econ Rev* 35: 519-530, 1946.

9. Geyman, JP. *Shredding the Social Contract: The Privatization of Medicare.* Monroe, ME. *Common Courage Press*, 2006, p. 206.

10. McCanne, D. Comment in quote-of-the-day on the November 2016 NBER Working Paper 22802, *National Bureau of Economic Research*, Cambridge, MA, November 7, 2016.

11. U. S. Department of Commerce. *The National Income and Products Accounts of the United States, 192901082L Statistical Tables, Table 6.21B.* Washington, DC : U.S. Department of Commerce.

12. Starr, P. *The Social Transformation of American Medicine.* New York. *Basic Books*, 1982, p. 448.

13. Commerce Department, Service Annual Survey 2016 or most recent available date for share of establishments.

14. Relman, AS. The new medical-industrial complex. *N Engl J Med* 303: 963-970, 1980.

15. Terhune, C. Health care in America: An employment bonanza and a runaway-cost crisis. *Kaiser Health News*, April 24, 2017.

16. Himmelstein, DU, Woolhandler, S. The current and projected taxpayer shares of U. S. health costs. *Amer J Public Health* online, January 21, 2016.

17. Geyman, JP. *Hijacked: The Road to Single Payer in the Aftermath of Stolen Health Care Reform.* Friday Harbor, WA. *Copernicus Healthcare*, 2010, pp. 7-36.

18. Herbert, B. This is reform? *New York Times*, August 17, 2009.

19. Field, RI. *Mother of Invention: How the Government Created "Free-Market" Health Care.* New York. *Oxford University Press*, 2014, pp. 220-221.

20. Suennen, L. Here come the exchanges . . . And the opportunity to turn chaos into gold. *Venture Valkyrie*, October 6, 2013.

21. Soltas, E. Nobody should get rich off Obamacare. *Bloomberg View*, December 3, 2013.

22. Metz, S. Reducing health care costs: delivery vs. financing approaches. *Health Care Disconnects*, November 12, 2013 (available at www.copernicus-healthcare.org)

23. National Institute for Health Care Management. A comparatively small number of sick people account for most health care spending. August 2, 2012.

24. Murphy, T. Aetna trumps 2Q expectations after scaling back ACA coverage. *ABC News*, August 3, 2017.

25. Johnson, C. Aetna chief executive says Obamacare is in a 'death spiral.' *The Washington Post*, February 15, 2017.

26. Potter, W. It's way past time for us to stop deluding ourselves about private health insurers. *The Progressive Populist*, September 1, 2016, p. 20.

27. Price, T, as quoted in Access to buying insurance is not health coverage. *Common Dreams*, January 19, 2017.

28. Hacker, JB. Why an open market won't repair American health care. *New York Times*, April 4, 2017.

29. Frum, D. *Trumpocracy: The Corruption of the American Republic.* New York. *HarperCollins*, 2018, p. 235.

30. Chomsky, N. As quoted by Polychroniou, CJ. Socialism for the rich, capitalism for the poor: An interview with Noam Chomsky. *Truthout*, December 16, 2016.

CHAPTER 2

HEALTH CARE POLICY: FOR SALE
TO THE HIGHEST BIDDER

This is not a new problem, as TR found more than 100 years ago and as FDR noted in his famous re-election speech in 1936:

Moneyed interests had begun to think of the Government of the United States as a mere appendage to their own affairs. We know that government by organized money is as dangerous as Government by organized mob. [1]

But today, arguably, this problem is the worst it has ever been and now threatens the survival of our supposed democracy.

This chapter has four goals: (1) to review the more recent history of the surge of outside money in the political process that has largely cancelled out the votes of many Americans; (2) to describe PhRMA, the pharmaceutical industry's trade group, as a poster child for this problem; (3) to consider how health policy and health care reform were subverted in the run-up to the ACA a decade ago; and (4) to briefly discuss the current health care debate in the aftermath of the GOP's failure to repeal and replace the ACA, despite having control of the White House and both chambers of Congress.

Surge of Money into Politics

Figure 2.1 gives us graphic evidence that outside spending in presidential and congressional year elections has skyrocketed over the last 25 years, accelerated especially after the Citizens United case of 2010, when the Supreme Court declared that corporations have the same constitutional rights as real people do, and that corporate spending on politics amounts to "speech" that is protected by the First Amendment. Shortly after that ruling, the 2010 *Speech Now* case ruled that supposedly "independent" expenditures to help a political candidate cannot be regulated at all. [2]

FIGURE 2.1

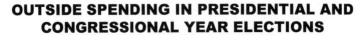

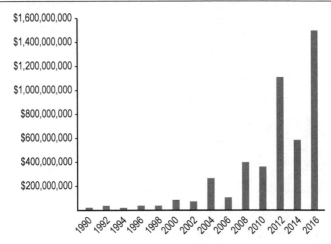

Spending by unrestricted political action groups (super PACs) and other unffiliated groups calculated in constant 2006 Dollars

Source: Center for Responsive Politics 2017

Figure 2.2 shows annual lobbying on health care in the last 20 years, with 2017 only a partial year.

Table 2.1 lists donations for members of the 115th Congress in 2017, with many of these names closely involved in crafting health care legislation.

FIGURE 2.2

ANNUAL LOBBYING ON HEALTH

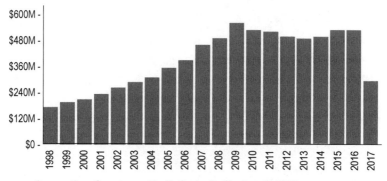

Source: OpenSecrets.org, Health Sector Profile, Aug. 7, 2017.

TABLE 2.1

DONATIONS TO MEMBERS OF THE 115TH
CONGRESS FROM THE HEALTH SECTOR, 2017

Sen. Mitch McConnell (R-KY)	$3,667,264
Sen. Orrin Hatch (R-UT)	$3,355,661
Sen. Charles Schumer (D-NY)	$2,715,088
Sen. Ron Wyden (D-OR)	$2,574,215
Sen. John Cornyn (R-TX)	$2,480,031
Sen. Roy Blunt (R-MISSOURI)	$2,409,872
Sen. Richard Burr (R-NC)	$2,289,736
Sen. Pat Toomey (R-PA)	$2,151,128
Sen. Rob Portman (R-OH)	$2,142,106
Sen. Bill Cassidy (R-LA)	$2,103,392
Rep. Paul Ryan (R-WI)	$1,943,669
Sen. Michael F. Bennett (D-CO)	$1,898,702
Sen. Marco Rubio (R-FL)	$1,781,409
Sen. Bob Casey (D-PA)	$1,744,516
Sen. Lamar Alexander (R-TN)	$1,725,507
Sen. Patty Murray (D-WA)	$1,698,733
Sen. Robert Menendez (D-NJ)	$1,667,151
Sen. Debbie Stabenow (D-MI)	$1,614,073
Sen. John Barrasso (R-WY)	$1,575,226
Sen. Sherrod Brown (D-OH)	$1,556,500

Source: Center for Responsive Politics, Washington, D.C.

If we think that legislators respond to the needs of their constituents more than to these contributions and the pressures from lobbyists as the main influences on legislation, Figure 2.3 dispels that notion in both parties.

FIGURE 2.3

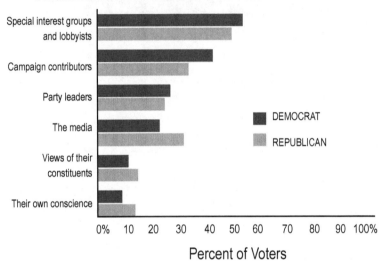

WHO DOES CONGRESS LISTEN TO?
constituents rank themselves near the bottom of the list

There are many examples of members of Congress taking money from special interests that directly influence their legislative behavior. Here are just three:

- Senator Ted Cruz (R-TX), who took in at least $3 million in outside funding in 2012, introduced a bill to allow mega donors and special interests to give unlimited contributions directly to candidates. He has said that "money absolutely can be speech," and that campaign financing reform was about "silencing" citizens.

- Rep. Darrell Issa (R-CA), one of the wealthiest members of Congress who just recently decided not to run for re-election, sponsored a bill to protect his top campaign contributors, government contractors, from having to disclose political spending.
- Rep. Ryan Costello (R-PA), who has received more than $300,000 in contributions from the drug industry over his career, has voted against any campaign finance reform bill and co-sponsored a bill that contributed to the opioid crisis by making it "virtually impossible" for the Drug Enforcement Agency to freeze suspicious shipments of drugs. [3]

The very wealthy oppose government's role in helping ordinary Americans, according to polls of multimillionaires, people in the top 1 or 2 percent by wealth. Examples: 61 percent majority of the American public support NHI financed by tax money vs. just 32 percent of the super wealthy; 68 percent of Americans believe that government must assure that nobody is without food, clothing and shelter vs. 43 percent of the multimillionaires. [4]

PhRMA as the Poster Child for Profiteering and Corruption

Together with another trade group, the Biotechnology Innovation Organization, PhRMA (The Pharmaceutical Research and Manufacturers of America) set a new record for lobbying the federal government in 2017—almost $35 million. They were trying to protect themselves from any crackdown on drug pricing as well as any adverse impacts from the tax overhaul bill.[5] PhRMA and its leading drug manufacturers have spent $1.8 billion on lobbying the federal government since 1999, according to the Center for

Responsive Politics. These funds are carefully targeted to lawmakers, their staffers and regulators involving legislation either favorable or problematic to their interests. Daniel Auble, who tracks lobbying activity for the Center for Responsive Politics, had this to say after some 1,500 lobbyists swarmed Capitol Hill promoting passage of the 21st Century Cures Act in 2016:

> *[This Act] is emblematic of the way laws get passed in Washington today: money is power, and no sector has more of both than the pharmaceutical industry.* [6]

In their ongoing attempts to retain their ability to set drug prices and avoid price controls, drug makers give money widely trying to defend their practices and gain friends and influence. As examples, PhRMA paid $14.3 million to think tanks, disease advocacy groups and universities in 2015 [7], while Pfizer gave $1 million to help finance Trump's inauguration. [8]

The ties between the pharmaceutical industry and the federal government have been deepening for years, including through revolving doors *in both directions*—to and from Congress and the Department of Health and Human Services (DHHS). Almost 340 former congressional staffers now work for drug companies or their lobbying firms, according to Legistorm, a nonpartisan congressional research company. Those who go from drug companies to staff jobs on Capitol Hill often are able to maintain their drug industry pensions and stock, according to *Kaiser Health News*. [9]

Conflicts of interest are common within the revolving doors between industry, K street, and the government. Consider these examples:

- Dr. Tom Price (R-GA), while chairing the House Budget Committee, sitting on the House Ways and Means Committee, and with a history of contacting the FDA on behalf of industry donors, invested in a sweetheart deal in a new drug targeting the U. S. market by a tiny biotech firm Innate Immunotherapeutics. That investment went up by 400 percent. House financial disclosures require reporting of ranges of value, not specific amounts. [10] As we know, he was Trump's first nominee to head DHHS, but was forced to resign as Secretary after disclosure of his use of private charter flights costing taxpayers more than $400,000. [11]

- Alex Azar, Trump's second appointee to head DHHS, pocketed almost $2 million in compensation during his final year as president of drug giant Eli Lilly's U. S. operations, plus another $1.6 million in severance pay and as much as $1 million from sale of his Eli Lilly stock. [12] During his tenure at Lilly, he presided over enormous price increases of Humalog insulin, which more than doubled between 2011 and 2016. [13] While at Lilly in 2009, he also helped to manage the fallout when Lilly paid a criminal fine of more than half a billion dollars to settle accusations that it had promoted Zyprexa, an anti-psychotic drug, for uses not approved by the FDA. [14]

PhRMA also targets state legislators with its lobbying efforts. A recent example is the industry's flooding the Louisiana state legislature with two lobbyists for every legislator to avoid passage of a bill that would require sales reps promoting medicines at physicians' offices to also reveal their prices. [15] PhRMA also gives big money to national political groups financing presidential, congressional, and state candidates, as well as patient advocacy groups for certain diseases. [16]

Price gouging is rampant throughout the drug industry. The industry typically defends large price increases as required to offset its costs of bringing new drugs to market, which on its face is disingenuous. The industry wildly exaggerates the costs of bringing a new drug to market, with most of its claimed R & D costs being marketing and non-rigorous trials conducted by drug companies themselves. They continue to lobby for accelerated approval of new drugs by the FDA with lesser evidence for efficacy.

These examples of price gouging have generated growing public outrage against the industry:

- When Gilead began marketing its new drug, Sovaldi, as a cure for the common hepatitis C liver virus, it was priced at $1,000 a pill, thereby costing $84,000 for a twelve-week treatment course. [17]

- The price of Lomustine, a drug for brain tumors and Hodgkin's lymphoma, has increased by almost 1,400 percent over the last four years, while the price of Daraprim, often used by patients with HIV, skyrocketed by about 5,500 percent from $13.50 to $750 per tablet in 2015. Martin Shkreli, founder and former CEO of Turing Pharmaceuticals, which manufactures Daraprim, was later found guilty on two counts of securities fraud. [18]

- The price of Mylan's EpiPen, a lifesaving treatment for emergency allergic reactions, increased by more than six-fold in several years to more than $300 per Epi-Pen; it is another example of a company buying an old drug, raising its price, and restricting patient access to a life-saving treatment.[19]

- The price of two pills of albendazole, a drug for hookworm, can cost as much as $400 in the U. S. vs. just 4 cents in Tanzania. [20]
- The prices of generic drugs are also soaring, partly as a result of industry consolidation and production slowdowns.[21]

According to a recent report from the U. S. Government Accountability Office, about two-thirds of drug companies have seen their profit margins increase by an average of 17 percent between 2006 and 2015. As Scott Knoer, chief pharmacy officer at Cleveland Clinic, observes:

Drug companies raise prices far exceeding inflation because they can. In the absence of regulation and without consumer awareness—since consumers don't generally see the price due to insurance—the sky is the limit. Ultimately, all of these costs are passed on to the government, insurance companies, patients and taxpayers. [22]

A recent report by National Academies of Sciences, Engineering, and Medicine, *Making Medicines Affordable: A National Imperative*, found that the U. S. pharmaceutical market is unsustainable and needs to change. Norman Augustine, chair of the study group, has this to say about the problem:

Drugs that are not affordable are of little value and drugs that do not exist are of no value. [23]

In his January State of the Union address to Congress, President Trump called reducing prescription drug prices one of his "greatest priorities," adding that "prices will come down." [24] This will almost certainly be just another lie and broken promise, not because of the enormous political power of PhRMA, but also because of the opposition of Alex Azar as head of DHHS to negotiated drug prices by Medicare [25], as the VA has done for many years, effectively reducing the prices of prescription drugs by about 42 percent. But we needn't hold our breath about significant change soon, despite passionate calls for action by hospitals, physicians, insurers, and patients. There is little consensus about how to solve the problem and continued inaction in Congress. [26]

We can see how the pharmaceutical industry is a good example of how corporate money and lobbying infiltrate government and dominate politics against the public interest. As a result, we have lost much of our supposed democratic process. As Wendell Potter and Nick Penniman say in their new book, *Nation on the Take: How Big Money Corrupts Our Democracy and What We Can Do About It*:

> *Our grand 240-year-old project of self-government has been derailed, replaced by a coin-operated system that mainly favors those who can pay to play.* [27]

How Outside Money Corrupted the ACA: 2008-2010

The Big Four—insurance industry, PhRMA, hospital industry, and the AMA— were the major players in the intense debate leading up to the passage of the ACA in 2010, but they were not the only ones. There were also many other players in the medical-industrial complex, ranging from the medical device and equipment industries to nursing homes and information technology. All wanted a seat at the table as competing bills moved forward in Congress. General Electric, as one example, then the 12th largest corporation in the world, had a big market share for imaging equipment and information technology. At that time, there were some 3,300 lobbyists in Washington D.C. spending $1.4 million a day lobbying for the special interests of these groups. [28]

These players were both defending their turfs and trying to expand their share of an expanded revenue pie to come under the guise of supporting reform. There was a blame game going on among these corporate interests as to who was responsible for the continued soaring costs of health care. As examples, insurers pointed to overcharging by hospitals, drug companies and physicians that left them no choice but to raise their premiums. Hospitals blamed physicians demanding higher payments as well as their rising burden of care for the uninsured and low reimbursement from Medicare and Medicaid. Robert Laszewski, president of the consulting firm Health Policy & Strategy Associates, noted:

It's always someone else's fault. There is not an incentive for these people to cooperate because the game they are playing is getting a bigger piece of the pie. [29]

There were conflicting interests and goals not only between these major players, but also within each group. As one example, a revolt took place within PhRMA that forced Billy Tauzin out from his $2 million a year job as CEO and head lobbyist, when he was perceived as too willing to bargain away the industry's profits and being too supportive of reform. [30]

The hospital industry was divided against itself, such as by divisions between urban and rural hospitals and between general and specialty hospitals.

Along the way in this contentious debate, there was some concern whether these corporate interests could forge a consensus. Finally voluntary, unenforceable pledges were made by the Big Four, which was soon labeled a "corporate alliance." Table 2.2 summarizes the pledges, agendas, tactics, and likely rewards for the Big Four stakeholders. [31] It is important to realize, however, that the public

TABLE 2.2

CORPORATE "ALLIANCE" FOR HEALTH CARE REFORM - THE BIG FOUR

Insurance Industry

Pledge	Abandon pre-existing conditions as an underwriting principle
	Accept all applicants
	Stop charging women higher premiums than men
Agenda	Grow private and public insurance markets by up to 50 million enrollees
Tactics	Oppose controls or caps on premium rates
	Oppose the public option
	Lobby for low standards for insurance coverage and low MLRs
	Fight against cuts of overpayments for Medicare Advantage plans
Rewards	Larger private and public markets
	Higher profits and returns to shareholders
	Preempt increased regulation by government

PhRMA

Pledge	$80 billion over 10 years toward costs of health care reform
Agenda	Expand private and public markets
	Avoid price controls and competition from importation of drugs from other countries
	Gain maximal patent protection for biotech drugs
Tactics	With assurance from White House agreement that government would not negotiate drug prices or import drugs from abroad, lobbied jointly with Families USA in support of health care reform as represented by bills in Congress
Rewards	Expanded private and public markets
	Higher profits and returns to shareholders
	Avoid increased regulation by government

Hospital Industry

Pledge	$155 billion over 10 years in reduced hospital charges
Agenda	Growth in future revenues in private and public markets
Tactics	Lobby for employer and individual mandates, and expansion of Medicaid
Rewards	Larger private and public markets
	Increased revenues ($170 billion), more than offsetting its pledged amount (40)

Organized Medicine

Pledge	No specific pledge
Agenda	Support private markets and restrain government intervention
	Prevent cuts in Medicare reimbursement
Tactics	Supports employer and individual mandates, insurance reforms, and expansion of Medicaid
	Opposes public option, rate-setting by independent commission, and targeted reimbursement cuts by specialty
Rewards	$245 billion "doc fix" restores Medicare reimbursement, at least for a time
	Increased revenues from expanded insured population

interest was left out of these negotiations, and that the revenues being sought by corporate stakeholders would become *our* costs as patients and taxpayers.

It became clear that the only way that corporate players could come to consensus would be if their investors would win. Indeed, Wall Street followed these negotiations closely, since the health care industry accounted for one-sixth of our economy. The insurance industry opposed the public option all along. When the Obama administration signaled its willingness to consider alternatives to a public plan, health insurer stocks were pushed higher despite a triple-digit loss in the broader markets. Trading in UnitedHealth and WellPoint jumped by about three-fold as investors placed calls and puts. [32]

Health care industries targeted both political parties in lobbying for their special interests. According to the Center for Public Integrity, by 2009 there were more than 4,500 lobbyists—eight for every member of Congress—attempting to influence the legislation. The lobbying industry had taken in $1.2 *billion* by the time the bill was passed. [33] As Bill Allison, a senior fellow at the Sunshine Foundation, said:

When you have a big piece of legislation like this, it's like ringing the dinner bell for K Street . . . There's a lot of money at stake and there are a lot of special interests who don't want their ox gored. [34]

Meanwhile, of course, in this uncertain political climate, corporate stakeholders in our profitable market-based system continue to throw big money to legislators on a bipartisan basis. As Benjamin Page, professor of decision-making at Northwestern University, and Martin Gilens, professor of politics at Princeton University, tell us in their new book, *Democracy in America? What Has Gone Wrong and What Can We Do About It*:

> *We believe that both major parties tend to be corrupted—and pushed away from satisfying the needs and wishes of ordinary Americans—by their reliance on wealthy contributors. We see this reliance as one of the major reasons for today's feeble state of democratic responsiveness. It is one of the main reasons that so many Americans are so angry at politicians. No wonder most Americans tell pollsters that public officials "don't care much what people like me think."* [35]

Concluding comment

This is where we are today: challenging whether we can reform health care. Keep this in mind as we go to the next chapters on TrumpCare, which show how far we are from what Teddy called a "square deal."

> *America's last Gilded Age gave rise to rebellious fires, the flames of which eventually spread to Teddy, a well-to-do Republican and progressive who was the single greatest champion of campaign finance reform this country has ever seen. He didn't believe in reform as an end in itself. He saw it as a means to reclaim the right to self-government, and the right for every person to have an equal opportunity to get ahead in life—what he termed a 'square deal.'* [36]

We will discuss a number of efforts to reverse Citizens United and restore American democracy in the last chapter of this book. But for now, it is time to proceed to the next five chapters that will describe what TrumpCare has brought us through its continued sabotage of the ACA.

References:

1. Roosevelt, FD. As quoted by Williams, BW. *Compromised: The Affordable Care Act and Politics of Defeat.* North Charleston, SC. *CreateSpace Independent Publishing Platform*, 2014, p. 9.

2. Page, BI, Gilens, M. *Democracy in America: What Has Gone Wrong and What We Can Do About It.* Chicago. *University of Chicago*, 2017, p. 187.

3. Big Money 20, *End Citizens United*, January, 2018.

4. Ibid#2, pp. 114-115.

5. Robbins, R. The drug industry's two big trade groups set a new record for lobbying in 2017. *STAT*, January 23, 2018.

6. Thebault, R. Big PhRMA's army of lobbyists. *Tarbell*, November 14, 2017.

7. Barrett, R. Drug industry association gives millions, gains friends. *Tarbell*, November 14, 2017.

8. Hancock, J, Lupkin, S, Lucas, E. With drug costs in crosshairs, health firms gave generously to Trump's inauguration. *Kaiser Health News*, April 19, 2017.

9. Lupkin, S. Big PhRMA greets hundreds of ex-federal workers at the 'revolving door.' *Kaiser Health News*, January 25, 2018.

10. Hancock, J, Bluth, R. Trump's DHHS nominee got a sweetheart deal from a foreign tech firm. *Kaiser Health News*, January 13, 2017.

11. Eilperin, J, Goldstein, A, Wagner, J. DHHS Secretary Tom Price resigns amid criticism for taking charter flights at taxpayer expense. *The Washington Post*, September 29, 2017.

12. Cancryn, A. Azar received millions from Eli Lilly in last year, disclosures show. *Politico*, November 20, 2017.

13. Armour, S, Radnovsky, L. Ex-Eli Lilly official is picked to run DHHS. *Wall Street Journal*, November 14, 2017.

14. Pear, R. Health nominee grilled on commitment to lower drug prices. *New York Times*, November 29, 2017.

15. Hancock, J, Luthra, S. As states target high drug prices, PhRMA targets state lawmakers. *Kaiser Health News*, February 1, 2027.

16. Hancock, J. Drug industry spent millions to squelch talk about high drug prices. *Kaiser Health News*, December 19, 2017.

17. Brill, S. *America's Bitter Pill: Money, Politics, Backroom Deals, and the Fight to Fix Our Broken Healthcare System*. New York. *Random House*, 2015, p. 449.

18. Emett, A. Big PhRMA raises price of cancer drug by 1,400 percent. *Nation of Change*, December 28, 2017.

19. Court, E. Mylan's epi-pen price increases are Valeant-like in size, Shkreli-like in approach. *Marketwatch*, August 18, 2016.

20. Whitehead, N. Why a pill that's 4 cents in Tanzania costs up to $400 in the U. S. *NPR*, December 11, 2017.

21. Associated Press. Soaring generic drug prices draw Senate scrutiny, November 20, 2014.

22. Kacik, A. Drug prices rise as PhRMA profit soars. *Modern Healthcare*, December 29, 2017.

23. Tribble, SJ. Experts tell Congress how to cut drug prices. We give you some odds. *California Healthline*, December 12, 2017.

24. Luthi, S. Reducing drug prices one of Trump's 'greatest priorities.' *Modern Healthcare*, February 1, 2017.

25. Ibid # 12.

26. Mershon, E. Among those who want to lower drug prices, there's cacophony, not consensus. *STAT*, January 26, 2018.

27. Potter, W, Penniman, N. *Nation on the Take: How Big Money Corrupts Our Democracy and What We Can Do About It*. New York. *Bloomsbury Press*, 2016, ix.

28. Adamy, J, Williamson, E. As Congress goes to break, health lobbying heats up. *Wall Street Journal*, August 5, 2009: A1.

29. Johnson, A. Race to pin blame for health costs. *Wall Street Journal*, February 5, 2010: A5.

30. Kirkpatrick, DD, Wilson, D. One grand deal to many costs Tauzin his job. *New York Times*, February 10, 2010: B1.

31. Geyman, JP. *Hijacked: The Road to Single Payer in the Aftermath of Stolen Health Care Reform*. Friday Harbor, WA. *Copernicus Healthcare*, 2010, p. 30.

32. Tracy, T. UnitedHealth, Aetna, WellPoint get bullish signal. *Wall Street Journal*, August 18, 2009: C3.

33. Center for Public Integrity, as cited by Moyers, B, Winship, M. The unbearable lightness of reform. *Truthout*, March 27, 2010.

34. Salant, JD, O'Leary, L. Six lobbyists per lawmaker work on health overhaul. *Bloomberg News*, as cited in *Truthout*, August 17, 2009.

35. Ibid #2, p. 111.

36. Roosevelt, TR. As quoted by Potter, W, Penniman, N. *Nation on the Take: How Big Money Corrupts Our Democracy and What We Can Do About It.* New York. *Bloomsbury Press*, 2016, p. 228.

What is TrumpCare?

*Oh, what a tangled web we weave
when first we practice to deceive.*

—Sir Walter Scott

CHAPTER 3

HOW TRUMPCARE OWNS THE
SABOTAGED AFFORDABLE CARE ACT

No one will lose coverage. There will be insurance for everybody.

—President Donald Trump,
promise on March 13, 2017. [1]

As we have already seen, the Trump administration and Republican controlled Congress, given the opportunity after the 2016 elections, failed completely on multiple occasions to repeal and replace the ACA. They also exposed to the world that they have no replacement plan. Instead they have launched a relentless campaign to dismantle the ACA, especially through administrative means. As economist Paul Krugman, *New York Times* Op-Ed columnist and Nobel laureate in economics, observes:

Now the government is run by people who couldn't repeal ObamaCare, but would clearly still like to see it fail—if only to justify the repeated, dishonest claims, especially by the tweeter in chief himself, that it was already failing. Or to put it differently, when Trump threatens to 'let ObamaCare fail,' what he's really threatening is to make it fail. [2]

This chapter has three goals: (1) to summarize the many ways whereby the ACA has been taken apart to the extent that it should now be called TrumpCare; (2) to show how the Trump administration and the Republican party own what they have wrought without congressional action and without broad political support among voters; and (3) to briefly describe some of the new directions that we can expect as TrumpCare further takes apart our current system.

Dismantling of Obamacare (ACA) by the GOP

Trump's first appointee to head DHHS was Dr. Tom Price, a Georgia multimillionaire and orthopedic surgeon. He was a long-time member of an alternative medical group that opposes Medicare, the ACA as a governmental intrusion into health care, and mandatory vaccination as "equivalent to human experimentation," and was a good fit for the Trump agenda for health care. Until he was forced to resign because of extensive use of charter flights at taxpayer expense exceeding $400,000, he presided over a number of ways to sabotage the ACA. [3] The enrollment window to sign up for the ACA was shortened from 90 to 45 days, federal spending to advertise the program was cut by 90 percent, and grants to organizations that help individuals sign up for coverage was chopped by 40 percent. For the first time, the federal government stopped promoting the ACA's website through television ads. This approach was based on a GOP theory that the fewer people enrolled in the ACA, the less the constituency to save it.[4] These changes did not come soon enough to affect the 2018 open-enrollment ACA signups, but will likely be in place during the 2018 signups for 2019.

In mid-October, Trump issued an Executive Order with many procedures intended to dismantle the ACA. Governmental agencies, including the Departments of Health and Human Services, Labor, and Treasury, were ordered to loosen restrictions on selling low-cost, short-term health insurance and association health plans; encourage tax-free employer contributions through health reimbursement accounts (HRAs); and propose other ways to increase choice and reduce consolidation in the health care market. Short-term plans can skirt the ACA's requirements to cover pre-existing conditions and provide coverage for essential health benefits, so that such benefits as hospitalization, maternity care, or prescription drugs would not have to be covered. At the same time, CSRs were discontinued, causing new uncertainties throughout the insurance industry.

Concerning the impacts of these changes, Kevin Lucia, a research professor at Georgetown's Health Policy Institute, warned that:

> *The combination of allowing less-regulated association plans, making it easier for employers to send workers to buy their own coverage and making short-term plans more broadly available is a concerted effort to undermine the individual market by drawing out the healthiest consumers.* [5]

Catherine Rampell, Op-Ed writer for *The Washington Post*, added this spot-on observation:

> *Somehow I don't remember [Trump] promising stadiums of cheering fans that he'd taken away protections for preexisting conditions, increased deductibles, spiked premiums, elimination of basic coverage requirements and, more generally, destabilization of the individual health insurance market.* [6]

At the end of October, Seema Verma, director of CMS, proposed a wide-ranging 365-page rule granting more flexibility and responsibility for health care to the states. Under the guise of "stabilizing insurance markets and allowing states and consumers more choice of plans," the rule allows states to decide how essential benefits should be defined, lets insurers spend more of premium dollars on administration and profits, and relaxed the threshold for state regulators to review premium increases from 10 to 15 percent.[7] More recent moves by CMS include the use of state waivers letting states establish work requirements for Medicaid beneficiaries, capping the years of Medicaid coverage, using drug screening to determine eligibility, and setting premiums that are unaffordable for low-income people. The work requirement is based on the false notion that patients needing Medicaid are too lazy to work and that these changes will somehow encourage them to get work and lift themselves out of poverty. As Verma disingenuously stated:

> *We owe our fellow citizens more than just handing them a Medicaid card. We owe a card with care. And more importantly, a card with hope.* [8]

The single biggest action to destroy the ACA, of course, was repeal of the individual mandate as part of the 2017 GOP tax cut bill passed by Congress at year's end. The accompanying tax penalty will be discontinued starting in 2019. Without the individual mandate, the CBO predicted that 13 million more Americans will drop or lose health insurance and that premiums will increase by about 10 percent annually on top of expected increases. [9]

How Trump and the GOP Own TrumpCare

Responding to Trump's termination of CSRs, House and Senate Minority Leaders Nancy Pelosi of California and Chuck Schumer of New York issued this joint statement:

> *It is a spiteful act of vast, pointless sabotage leveled at working families and the middle class in every corner of America. Make no mistake about it, Trump will try to blame the Affordable Care Act, but this will fall on his back and he will pay the price for it.* [10]

Senator Lindsey Graham (R-SC) had this to say after the individual mandate was repealed:

Once you've repealed the individual mandate, politically, you own this thing. [11]

A November 2017 national poll by the Kaiser Family Foundation found that more than 60 percent of respondents believe that the Trump administration and congressional Republicans are responsible for any and all future problems with the sabotaged ACA. (Figure 3.1) [12] Commenting on an article in *The Washington Post* on Obamacare, Duane Bender called for a clear-cut name change of what this administration has brought us:

> *It's time for the press to stop calling the ACA "Obama Care." What's left of the ACA should now be referred to as TrumpCare, and Trump and the Republicans should be held accountable for all future premium increases and access issues. Young, healthy, well-employed people will give Trump credit for allowing them to pay less (or not at all) for health insurance. So he should also get the blame for the impact on the older, sicker, and poorer people caused by his actions.* [13]

People for the American Way concluded that the Senate's failed TrumpCare bills in 2017 would have these disastrous consequences:

1. The short-term cuts to Medicaid are painful.
2. The long-term cuts to Medicaid are far worse.
3. The uninsured population would rise in every age group ...
4. ... and in every state.
5. Premiums would jump, especially for the older and poorer.
6. Employer plans are not safe either.
7. Tax credits for the middle class would plummet.
8. Hospitals would bear a heavy burden.
9. It's a job killer. [14]

FIGURE 3.1

MOST SAY PRESIDENT TRUMP AND REPUBLICANS IN CONGRESS ARE RESPONSIBLE FOR ANY FUTURE PROBLEMS WITH THE ACA

As you may know, the 2010 health care law, also known as Obamacare, remains the law of the land. Which comes closer to your view?

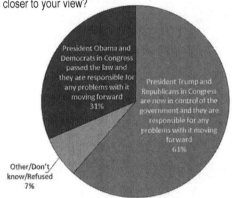

NOTE: "Other" incudes the shares that say "Neither of these/someone else is responsible" (Vol.) and "Both are equally responsible" (Vol.).
SOURCE: Kaiser Family Foundation Health Tracking Poll (conducted March 28-April 3, 2017)

As the Trump administration pursues further sabotage of the ACA, legal actions are being brought forward on a number of fronts. Eighteen state attorneys general and the District of Columbia sought an immediate restraining order to reinstate CSR payments, but a federal judge denied that petition within days. A lawsuit was brought by the GOP in the House in 2014 against the Obama administration asserting that these payments could not be made without congressional appropriation. That suit is still pending as insurers plead their case that these payments are needed to contain their costs and preserve coverage for enrollees at discounted rates. [15] A class action lawsuit is being proposed that challenges whether CMS has the authority to let states impose any premiums on low-income Medicaid enrollees. [16] Legal advocates challenge the legality of placing work requirements on Medicaid recipients, since that is beyond the current law and would require an act of Congress, not administrative policies. [17] A class action lawsuit has recently been filed against the Centene Corporation, the nation's largest Medicaid managed care plan, alleging that it is marketing junk plans with inadequate numbers of providers within their networks. [18]

New Directions under TrumpCare

Here are some of the major ways that TrumpCare will decrease access to health care in this country while failing to contain uncontrolled cost increases throughout our increasingly deregulated and privatized market-based "system."

1. Repeal of the individual mandate.

As we saw in the first chapter, we need the largest possible risk pool in order to have the most efficient system for health insurance. In order to contain costs for everyone, healthier people need to share the costs of sicker people. All of us will get sick or have a major accident requiring costly care at some points in our lives, much of it unpredictable.

The individual mandate was an attempt to bring younger, healthier people into a larger risk pool. Its loss will lead to insurers raising prices and exiting markets that are not sufficiently profitable, especially in rural areas, where costs are higher and providers fewer. It appears that 454 counties in the U. S. will have only one insurer in 2018, where the cheapest plan for a 40-year-old consumer will cost more than $500 a month, or $6,000 a year. [19] An increasing number of counties will have *no* insurers. As premiums become unaffordable for more and more people, it will lead to a vicious cycle of smaller, more segmented risk pools within which insurance costs more and provides less.

2. Discontinued cost sharing reduction (CSR) payments.

Trump's executive action in October of 2017 to terminate federal CSR payments to insurers caused more uncertainty and disruption within their markets. The CBO estimated that about 5 percent of people who had purchased their own coverage under the ACA marketplaces would have no insurers in 2018, and that premiums would rise by about 20 percent for the others. Private insurers, beholden as they are to their financial bottom lines and their shareholders, are now forced to recover the money lost by withheld CSRs, either by raising premiums sufficiently or leaving markets altogether. Those enrollees who still qualify for tax credits will not be affected, but about 7.5 million people who earn too much for these credits will have to decide whether they can still afford insurance. As he announced his decision to remove CSR payments, opposed by virtually all stakeholders within the health care system, Trump told us yet another lie:

> *This is promoting health care choice and competition all across the United States. This is going to be something that millions and millions of people will be signing up for, and they're going to be very happy.* [20]

3. State waivers

We can expect that state waivers under Section 1115 will become common as the federal government shifts responsibility for health care to the states. As head of CMS, Seema Verma is already presiding over these waivers, based on the supposed theory that:

> *We must allow states, which know the unique needs of their citizens, to design programs that don't merely provide a Medicaid card but provide care that allows people to rise out of poverty and no longer need public assistance. . . True*

compassion is lifting Americans most in need out of difficult circumstances. The new flexibility requested by states will allow them to partner with us to help program beneficiaries live healthy, fulfilling lives as independently as possible. . . . We owe it to these Americans to try whatever may help them achieve the dignity and self-sufficiency they deserve. [21]

With waivers in hand, states will be able to ignore the essential health benefits required by the ACA. We can expect to see insurers marketing such skinny policies as to not justify the word "insurance," but at attractive premiums that will lead enrollees to think they have coverage. That is, until they really need it with a major illness or accident. Work requirements have already been established for Medicaid enrollees in Kentucky and Indiana, with ten more states lined up to request the same. This approach ignores what we know about the extent to which Medicaid enrollees are already working. According to the Kaiser Family Foundation, almost 8 in 10 live in working families and a majority are working themselves, while many work part-time and can't find full-time work or have major impediments to being able to work. [22]

Lifetime caps on Medicaid coverage, ranging from three to five years, are being considered by Arizona, Kansas, Maine, Utah, and Wisconsin. Cost sharing with Medicaid beneficiaries is becoming more common, as shown in Figure 3.2. [23] In addition to its work requirement, Kentucky will lock people out of the program if premiums are not paid, and eliminate retroactive eligibility. [24] Other pending waivers include Arkansas' request to reduce its eligibility for enrollees under its expanded Medicaid program from 138 percent of federal poverty level to 100 percent, adopting a closed drug formulary excluding some medications, and elimination of presumptive eligibility for patients needing immediate care. Separately from the

FIGURE 3.2

CHARGING MEDICAID BENEFICIARIES

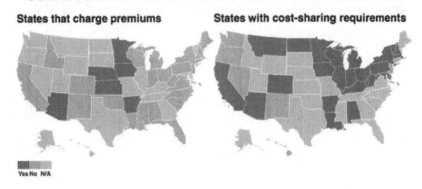

States that charge premiums   **States with cost-sharing requirements**

Yes No N/A

Source: Kaiser Family Foundation

1115 waivers, CMS is allowing states to exclude Planned Parenthood services. [25] All of these changes will get much worse as Medicaid cuts take effect under the new federal budget.

4. *Short-term plans*

Short-term health insurance has been a way for insurers to get around the constraints established by the ACA, such as requiring coverage of ten essential health benefits and banning denial of coverage due to preexisting conditions. A final rule released by the Trump administration in August 2018 relaxed all of the ACA's requirements for insurers, opening up a new market of less expensive plans up to one year that cover very little. Renewable for up to three years (unless enrollees develop a new deniable health condition), these plans typically set annual and lifetime benefits, do not have a standard set of benefits, and exclude coverage for preventive care, maternity care, pediatric services, dental care, rehabilitative services, substance abuse, and mental health services. With very limited coverage for prescription drugs, patients getting cancer face the burden of oncology drugs that average $10,000 a month. [26]

Short-term plans have lower premiums and deductibles than ACA plans and will be attractive to younger, healthier people. Though very profitable to insurers, these plans qualify for the term "junk insurance." Andy Slavitt, who headed CMS during the Obama administration, observed:

> *This is Trump's biggest assault to the ACA, American families, and the law. [After failing to repeal the ACA in 2017], 2018 Trump is just skipping the voting part and ignoring the law.* [27]

5. *Association health plans (AHPs)*

Republicans for years have favored the use of association health plans whereby small businesses can join associations that offer insurance to their members, typically across state lines. They have had problems in the past, such as providing little or no coverage for such services as chemotherapy or even doctor visits, insolvency, fraud, and lack of consumer protections. [28] Under a new rule just released by CMS, association health plans are likely to become more common under a deregulated TrumpCare. These plans will be marketed to employers as providing more affordable coverage starting in 2019 without complying with any of the ACA's requirements. They will be free to avoid coverage of some essential health benefits, and spend less than 80 percent of their premium revenue on administration and profits. They can be expected to expose enrollees to high out-of-pocket costs, siphon off healthier individuals for coverage, and further segment the insurance risk pool. [29]

Association health plans have a long history of fraud. The U. S. Government Accountability Office identified 144 "unauthorized or bogus" plans from 2000 to 2002. Jim Quiggle, spokesman for the Coalition Against Insurance Fraud, which includes the Blue

Cross and Blue Shield Association and the National Association of Insurance Commissioners, warns that:

> *The relaxed federal standards for forming AHPs risk opening the doors wider to a surge of scam operators who will seek to exploit the looser environment.* [30]

Despite the hype for AHPs by the Trump administration, they have not been well received by the business community. The National Federation of Independent Business (NFIB) recently decided against setting one up, describing the new Trump rules as unworkable. [31]

6. Health Savings Accounts (HSAs)

The GOP has for years touted HSA's as a way for people to put aside money, tax-free, to save for their future health care expenses. Currently, individuals can make these contributions up to $3,400 a year, or $6,750 for families. Those limits are likely to increase in the near future, but we know from experience that HSAs have failed, especially for lower-income people who cannot afford to put such money aside. Although the use of HSA's has increased dramatically in recent years (Figure 3.3), the benefits have gone to the wealthy and Wall Street, where they are managed. Although Republicans have long promoted the value of raising the annual limits for HSA contributions, it doesn't accomplish its purpose. A 2016 study found that less than one-half of people with HSAs deposited any money in them. [32] As Maura Calsyn, managing director of health policy at the Center for American Progress, observes:

> *Raising the limits is essentially just providing high-income individuals with a greater tax benefit and doesn't do anything to increase coverage.* [33]

FIGURE 3.3

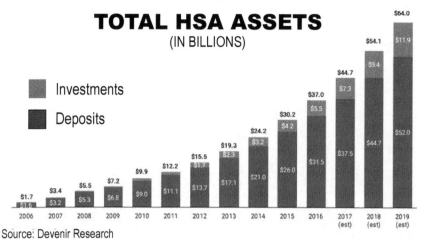

TOTAL HSA ASSETS
(IN BILLIONS)

- ■ Investments
- ■ Deposits

Source: Devenir Research

Although HSAs are not useful health policy for Americans in need, they have become a huge and very profitable industry on Wall Street, especially since the November 2016 elections. In the six months after the elections, the shares of HSA provider HealthEquity rose by about 35 percent to become one of the best performing stocks. Optum Bank, the industry leader, is owned by UnitedHealth Group, the nation's largest health insurer, and has more than 3 million accounts and $7 billion in assets that it manages for its clients. [34]

Overall, these directions are worse for patients and more profitable for corporate stakeholders in our runaway market-based system. We will see ongoing premium increases as insurance and health care become even less affordable, more cost-shifting to patients, decreasing access, less choice, worse patient outcomes, increasing bureaucracy and more counties without any insurers. We will also see further disruption of ACA sign-ups, confusion and uncertainty among the public, and problems with automatic re-enrollment ACA plans.

As these changes take place, the GOP and Trump will claim cost savings to the federal government while many states will be unable to bear their increased burden of providing care and any kind of a safety net. Health care, especially cuts to Medicare and Medicaid, will become a pawn in the debate over controlling the growing deficit that was caused by the tax giveaway to the wealthy by the recent tax "reform" bill.

Concluding comment

What we're seeing is an unprecedented shift of federal responsibility for health care to the states, which is a total breech of the social contract with Americans established more than 50 years ago with the passage of Medicare and Medicaid. President Lyndon Johnson signed the Social Security Amendments for Medicare and Medicaid on July 30, 1965 with the goal to "improve a wide range of health and medical services for Americans of all ages." These changes will be called into question in the courts in today's political environment, with "the heart of the matter, as always, being the question of how our nation views the core objectives of the Medicaid program—as health care or welfare for the nearly 70 million Americans enrolled." [35]

Richard Eskow, senior fellow at Campaign for America's Future, describes our present predicament this way:

> *Give them less and make them think it's more. That's the Republican Party's goal with "TrumpCare." Why? They're doing it to provide enormous tax breaks to the wealthiest among us, after we have already achieved levels of inequality not seen since the Roaring Twenties or the Gilded Age of the Nineteenth Century.* [36]

The states are less prepared for their new burdens than the federal government, as we shall see in the next chapter.

References:

1. Trump, DJ. As quoted by Jackson, HC. 6 promises Trump has made about health care. *Politico*, March 13, 2017.

2. Krugman, P. Health care in a time of sabotage. *New York Times*, July 21, 2017.

3. Eilperin, J. DHHS secretary resigns amid criticism for taking charter flights at taxpayer expense. *The Washington Post*, September 29, 2017.

4. Demko, P, Pradhan, R, Cancryn, A. Confusion clouds open enrollment with Republicans still eager to dismantle Obamacare. *Politico*, October 29, 2017.

5. Appleby, J. Trump's order advances GOP go-to ideas to broaden insurance choices, curb costs. *Kaiser Health News*, October 12, 2017.

6. Rampell, C. Trump's Obamacare order could destroy the health-care system. *The Washington Post*, October 12, 2017.

7. Meyer, H, Livingston, S, Dickson, V. CMS to allow states to define essential benefits. *Modern Healthcare*, October 29, 2017.

8. Verma, S, as quoted by Lighty, M. New Medicaid work requirements will deny more care. *Sanders Institute*, November 15, 2017.

9. Cunningham, PW. The Health 202: Your health policy appointment. *The Washington Post*, December 21, 2017.

10. Pelosi, N, Schumer, C. As quoted by the *Associated Press*. Trump to issue stop-payment order on health care subsidies, *New York Times*, October 13, 2017.

11. Graham, L., as quoted by Kenen, J. The stealth repeal of Obamacare. *Politico*, December 19, 2017.

12. Weixel, N. Poll: 60 percent to blame Trump, GOP for ObamaCare problems. *The Hill*, November 17, 2017.

13. Bender, D. As quoted as a comment on Rampell, C. Trump is hoping you won't notice backdoor repeal of Obamacare. *The Washington Post*, January 15, 2018.

14. Talking Points Memo (TPM): 9 devastating impacts of the Senate's TrumpCare bill.

15. Cunningham, PW. Here's one legal and political battle you didn't expect: Republicans versus health insurers. *The Washington Post*, January 10, 2018.

16. Meyer, H. Legal clash over Medicaid premiums could derail GOP rollback of expansion. *Modern Healthcare*, February 6, 2018.

17. Corcoran, M. A legal battle is mounting against the GOP's attack on Medicaid. *Truthout*, February 6, 2017.

18. Small, L. Centene slapped with lawsuit over provider networks in ACA exchange plans. *Fierce Healthcare*, January 12, 2018.

19. Levey, NN. Republicans' latest plan to repeal Obamacare's insurance requirement could wreak havoc in some very red states. *Los Angeles Times*, November 27, 2017.
20. Trump, DJ. As quoted by Rovner, J, Carey, MA, Appleby, J. Trump acting solo: What you need to know about changes to the health law. *Kaiser Health News*, October 13, 2017.
21. Verma, S. Making Medicaid a pathway out of poverty. *The Washington Post*, February 4, 2018.
22. Garfield, R, Rudowitz, R, Damico, A. Understanding the intersection of Medicaid and work. *Kaiser Family Foundation*, January 5, 2018.
23. Ibid # 16.
24. Rosenbaum, S, Wachino, V, Gunsalus, R et al. State 1115 proposals to reducing Medicaid eligibility: Assessing their scope and projected impact. *The Commonwealth Fund*, January 11, 2018.
25. Wynne, B, Cowey, T. State waivers as a national policy lever: The Trump administration, work requirements, and other potential reforms in Medicaid. *Health Affairs Blog*, February 6, 2018.
26. Appleby, J. Trump administration loosens restrictions on short-term health plans. *Kaiser Health News*, August 1, 2018.
27. Slavitt, A. As quoted by Corbett, J. Continuing sabotage of Americans' healthcare, Trump proposes allowing insurers to offer 'junk plans.' *Common Dreams*, February 20, 2018.
28. Appleby, J. Association health plans: A favorite GOP approach to coverage poised for comeback. *Kaiser Health News*, October 6, 2017.
29. Appleby, J. Trump administration rule paves way for association health plans. *Kaiser Health News*, January 4, 2018.
30. Quiggle, J. As quoted by Meyer, H. Fraud fears rise as feds expand access to association health plans. *Modern Healthcare*, June 21, 2018.
31. Cancryn, A. Trump promised them better, cheaper health care. It's not happening. *Politico*, July 19, 2018.
32. Andrews, M. GOP seeks to sweeten health savings account deals. Will consumers bite? *Kaiser Health News*, July 14, 2017.
33. Calsyn, M. As quoted by Appleby, J. HSAs: 'Tax-break trifecta' or insurance gimmick benefiting the wealthy? *Kaiser Health News*, February 3, 2017.
34. Terhune, C, Appleby, J. Companies behind health savings accounts could bank on big profits under GOP plan. *Kaiser Health News*, March 14, 2017.
35. Ibid # 25.
36. Eskow, RJ. GOP 'Health' Bill: Death, disaster, and Gilded Age greed. *Common Dreams*, June 23, 2017.

CHAPTER 4

SHIFTING HEALTH CARE
TO THE STATES

As we saw in the last chapter, the GOP and Trump administration are committed to shifting responsibility for health care from the federal government to the states through waivers to get around constraints of the ACA and through state block grants. Timothy Jost, J.D., professor emeritus of law at the Washington and Lee School of Law, brings us this important insight to better understand the Trump agenda for health care:

> *A state-based approach to health insurance reform is very attractive because it shifts the political and financial responsibility for coming up with an ACA replacement away from Congress to the states. Congress and the administration can say it is not our fault that millions are losing coverage—the states are to blame.* [1]

The Trump budget released in February 2018 for fiscal year 2019 gives us further evidence of his war on the poor and middle class. His proposal would cut the budget of DHHS by 20.3 percent, slash the budgets of Medicaid and Medicare by $1.3 trillion and $554 billion, respectively, and cut Social Security by $10 billion. [2] This budget represents just one more Trump lie, as the Editorial Board of the *New York Times* reports, noting that Trump tweeted in May

2015 that "I was the first and only potential GOP candidate to state there would be no cuts to Social Security, Medicare and Medicaid," and that he promised during the presidential campaign that he would "champion the forgotten men and women of our country." [3]

The Trump budget would also eliminate the expansion of Medicaid under the ACA and cut food stamps, converting them into a hybrid of commodity deliveries and cash benefits. [4] Budget cutbacks are also a big part of this strategy under the guise of cutting the federal deficit, which soared with the December 2017 "tax cut" bill (really a $1.5 trillion tax scam), which mostly cut taxes for the very wealthy.

This chapter has three goals: (1) to describe some of the many ways that states are avoiding the ACA's constraints, especially involving Medicaid; (2) to assess the likely effects of state block grants; and (3) to briefly consider the adverse impacts of state-based Medicaid under TrumpCare.

How States are Taking Medicaid Apart and Rendering the ACA Irrelevant

What to do about Medicaid is at the center of a battle royal in Congress and across the country. Thirty-one states expanded Medicaid under the ACA, and a 2018 referendum was passed in Maine adding that state to the list. Almost 75 million lower-income Americans are covered by Medicaid, with 73 percent in private Medicaid plans.

Here are some of the many ways that Medicaid will be devastated by TrumpCare, mostly through federal waivers as authorized by Seema Verma's 365-page rule in October 2017 giving states an "unprecedented level of flexibility" to design their Medicaid programs as they see fit." [5]

1. Eliminating the individual mandate

We are now seeing big differences in how states are reacting to the elimination of the individual mandate in the December 2017 tax bill. At least nine blue states, plus the District of Columbia, are pursuing initiatives to keep their own versions of the mandate in order to broaden the risk pool and make health insurance more affordable. [6] Red states welcome the absence of the individual mandate starting in 2019 when penalties will be removed if people are uninsured. There is, however, precedent for how well individual mandates can effectively keep more people insured. Massachusetts was the first state to require state residents to have health insurance, enacted in 2006, and it has the lowest rate of uninsured in the country—just 2.5 percent. [7]

2. Work requirements

Ten states—Arizona, Arkansas, Indiana, Kansas, Kentucky, Maine, New Hampshire, North Carolina, Utah, and Wisconsin—have already requested waivers to impose work requirements on their Medicaid enrollees, to begin in 2019. As one example, Kentucky will require Medicaid beneficiaries to work at least 80 hours a month. Exemptions will be made for the disabled, pregnancy, or being a primary caretaker. Indiana will exempt people over 60 years of age, and those who are chronically homeless or recently incarcerated. [8] In Mississippi, where eligibility for Medicaid is limited to annual income less than $5,000 and where 91 percent of Medicaid beneficiaries are mothers, they all lose eligibility if they work 20 hours a week at a minimum income wage. [9]

While CMS amazingly says that states will have to test whether the work requirement will improve enrollees' health, Judith Solomon, vice president of the Center on Budget and Policy Priorities, responds:

> *What health outcome will be improved if we take away*
> *health care from those not able to work.* [10]

3. Reducing essential benefits

The ACA requires insurers to cover these 10 essential
benefits without dollar caps: outpatient services; emergency services;
hospitalization; maternity and newborn care; mental health and
substance abuse disorder, including behavioral health treatment;
prescription drugs; rehabilitative and habilitative services and
devices; laboratory services; preventive and wellness services and
chronic disease management; and pediatric services, including oral
and vision care. Any of these can be excluded by new plans under
TrumpCare, as a way to lower premiums and render their "insurance"
less useful.

4. Income premiums that people won't be able to afford

The Healthy Indiana Plan has already shown how a premium
requirement for the poor is a serious barrier to care. As Joan Alker,
executive director of Georgetown University's Center for Children
and Families, notes:

> *The Healthy Indiana Plan has already shown how a*
> *premium requirement for the poor is a serious barrier to care.* [11]

Seniors are also especially vulnerable to this change, since they
can be charged five times what younger people will be charged.

5. Capping the years that enrollees can be on Medicaid.

Caps of three to five years are being considered in some states
without regard for peoples' needs.

6. Drug testing and basing eligibility on drug screening.

Some states, such as Wisconsin, are considering this approach as another way to reduce its enrollments on Medicaid. Other states are going right ahead on their own to challenge the authority of DHHS to enforce any aspects of the ACA. Idaho's Republican governor, C. L. Otter, has signed an executive order to combat what he called "the overreaching, intrusive nature of Obamacare" by allowing insurers to sell plans that do not comply with the ACA's requirements.

Alex Azar, the new head of DHHS, is confronted with a decision whether to enforce the ACA law or not, and so far has indicated only that "we'll be looking at that very carefully and measure it up against the standards of the law." [12] He sees the decision by the Idaho Department of Insurance to allow insurers to market non-ACA compliant plans as a "cry for help." [13] Blue Cross of Idaho already plans to market five new plans named *Freedom Blue* by April 2018 that break with the ACA is such ways as limiting coverage, setting dollar caps, varying premiums by a ratio of five to one based on age, and discriminating against applicants based on preexisting conditions. These approaches may well be challenged in the courts. [14]

All of these strategies to undercut the ACA's requirements through state waivers reduce access to care while also reducing Medicaid enrollments and thus states' spending on health care. Predictably, they also lead many people to forgo or delay necessary care and have worse outcomes. In Indiana, for example, where Seema Verma (now CMS head) implemented various cutbacks to Medicaid in her disingenuously named Healthy Indiana Plan 2.0, access to HIV prevention and drug treatment was restricted and has led to an opioid and HIV epidemic in parts of the state. Michael Lighty, Director of Public Policy for the California Nurses Association/National Nurses

United, brings us this important insight concerning the destruction of what has been a social contract with lower-income Americans' health care since 1965:

> *We cannot stand by and allow these new ways to deny care. There will likely be lawsuits and rightly so. In the case of the Roberts decision that limited the Medicaid expansion under Obamacare, such expansion has been left up to the states. That doesn't mean that the states should be free to simply impose requirements that have nothing to do with legitimate eligibility. Medicaid is too important a program to be exploited by a conservative social engineering agenda to punish out-of-work poor people in an economy that doesn't provide enough jobs— much less jobs that pay a living wage. Rather, Medicaid is a program to make sure that we have a basic level of care in this country.* [15]

Why State Block Grants Are a Bad Idea

Federal budget cutting of "entitlements" (read especially Medicaid) has been part of the GOP mantra for a long time, together with turning this program over to the states. The Graham-Cassidy bill, although it failed to pass Congress in 2017, may well turn up again in some form in 2018. It would have eliminated Obamacare's expansion of state Medicaid programs and let states apply for state block grants to design their own Medicaid programs over just a two-year period. As 15 Republican governors said in September 2017:

> *Adequately funded, flexible block grants to the states are the last, best hope to finally repeal and replace Obamacare.* [16]

Under these kinds of block grants, states would be free to use federal money in any number of ways, including direct payments to providers, subsidies for private insurers, high-risk pools, and removal of the ACA's constraints on insurers. Federal payments to the states for Medicaid would likely be capped. The new Trump budget would cut federal Medicaid spending by $675 billion by 2028, and is supported by Alex Azar, the new DHHS head. [17]

There are all kinds of problems with block grants to states. These are just some of them.

1. *Startup times are inadequate.*

It took Massachusetts every bit of four years to establish its program. Many states will not be up to the challenge of designing their own programs. State legislative calendars will be a problem— Texas' legislature, for example, will not convene until 2019!

2. *Obamacare coverage would disappear everywhere in 2020.*

States would be ineligible for more federal funding unless they have a plan and apply in time. Without a functioning new system, consumers and markets will be thrown into chaos. [18]

3. *State block grants would decimate Medicaid and end a more than 50-year social contract with poor and lower-income Americans.*

Many millions of people would lose any health insurance. State block grants would gut Medicaid, which covers about one-half of obstetric deliveries and two-thirds of nursing home costs. [19] Since two-thirds of nursing home costs are paid by Medicaid, some nursing homes will close. Where will all those patients go?

4. *Many essential health care services would no longer be covered.*

With less federal money in hand and more latitude to reduce coverage, states can opt to cut coverage for such essential services as hospitalization, prescription drugs, maternity care, and mental health services, or any others of the 10 essential benefits required by the ACA.

5. *Increasing premiums and cost sharing will reduce access to care.*

Since states would be free to set premiums and other forms of cost-sharing, we can expect that they will do so as they face inevitable pressures on their state budgets.

6. *Applicants for Medicaid will lose choice.*

Many insurers are already leaving markets viewed as not sufficiently profitable. Figure 4.1 shows the widespread number of U. S. counties with only one insurer in 2018.

Figure 4.1

U. S. COUNTIES PROJECTED TO HAVE JUST ONE INSURER IN 2018

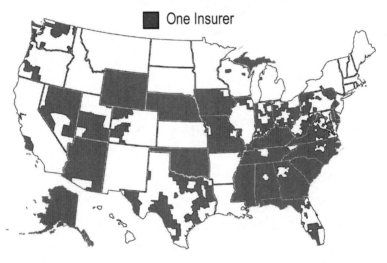

Source: Robert Wood Johnson Foundation

7. *Medicaid will continue as a grossly underfunded program seen as "welfare" by the GOP, not an essential safety net program.*

Caps of federal payments to the states for Medicaid will likely decrease over future years. The case of Puerto Rico shows us how bad this problem can be. A statutory cap of 50 percent was established there in 1968. By 2010, the federal share of Puerto Rico's Medicaid had dropped to just 18 percent. Nurse midwife services and long-term care are not covered today. A recent study of Medicaid caps led researchers to this conclusion:

> *States cannot afford the steep cuts in federal Medicaid spending—about $800 billion over 10 years amounting to a 24 percent reduction that would increase to 35 percent in the following decade—that House and Senate Republicans have proposed. Capped funding inevitably would force states to make painful decisions about reducing Medicaid eligibility and benefits. Medicaid funding caps would unravel the program in many states, leaving millions of low-income persons without any health insurance.* [20]

8. State block grants for Medicaid will end up as a gift to private insurers, who will take profits on the backs of the most vulnerable among us.

Insurers will be able to charge higher premiums before state regulators look at their hikes (those more than 15 percent). They will also be able to avoid the ACA's provision that has required them to spend at least 80 percent of their premium revenue on direct patient care. Instead, they can decrease what they call their "medical loss ratio," increase their own administrative and marketing costs and increase profits.

9. *Demonstration programs in states are inadequately evaluated.*

Almost three-quarters of states have Medicaid demonstration projects, such as testing whether enrollees should be required to pay premiums. These projects often account for a majority of a state's Medicaid budget and cost the federal government $300 billion a year. The GAO has found that states' evaluation of these projects under Section 1115 waivers are inadequate and that oversight by CMS has been lax. [21]

10. *We can learn from Canada's forty-year experience with block grants.*

Canada implemented a block grant policy to the provinces 40 years ago, with the hope that the provinces could reduce costs by improving the efficiency of care. Those hopes have not been achieved. Instead, provinces have been forced to reduce funding to hospitals and bargain harder with professional associations. If we don't learn from the Canadian experience, we will see more hospital closures and more physicians unwilling to see Medicaid patients because of even lower reimbursement policies than today. As two researchers concluded from their 2017 study of block grants in Canada:

> *The Canadian experience suggests that a block grant policy for Medicaid is most likely to succeed in only one aspect— reducing federal spending on the program. It would do so by shifting costs to states and forcing untenable trade-offs that would limit access to care for low-income U. S. residents.* [22]

Adverse Impacts of State-Based Medicaid under TrumpCare

The CBO has previously projected that 13 million people will lose health insurance with repeal of the individual mandate, which will go away under TrumpCare. Even if covered by Medicaid, that coverage will be fragile as enrollees are on again and off again, as coverage covers less care, as their choices diminish, and as cost sharing requirements force many to forgo or delay care. Worse outcomes will occur due to these delays as the numbers of preventable deaths increase.

States will find that premiums and cost sharing in Medicaid will not lead to significant savings. A recent study by the Kaiser Family Foundation came to these conclusions:

Even small levels of cost sharing in the range of $1 to $5 are associated with reduced use of care, including necessary services. State savings from premiums and cost sharing in Medicaid and the Children's Health Insurance Program (CHIP) are limited. Research shows that potential revenue gains from premiums and cost sharing are offset by increased disenrollment, increased use of more expensive services, such as emergency room care, and increased costs in other areas, such as resources for uninsured individuals and administrative expenses. [23]

Community health centers, a backbone for primary care across the country, will lose funding, as will hospitals, nursing homes, and other safety net programs, such as CHIP and the Supplemental Nutrition Assistance Program (SNAP) (food stamps) because of lack of funds at the state level. The American Association of Retired Persons (AARP) has taken this strong stand against state block grants for Medicaid:

AARP opposes Medicaid block grants and per capita caps because we are concerned that such proposals will endanger the health, safety, and care of millions of individuals who depend on the essential services provided through Medicaid. [24]

The impacts of state-based Medicaid will be especially harsh on rural areas, both for patients and hospitals that depend on insured patients. There have already been 83 rural hospital closures since 2010, resulting in restricted access to lifesaving services, maternity care, and care for chronic conditions. In addition, these closures result in loss of many jobs, since rural hospitals are often the largest employer in the community. [25]

David Blumenthal, president of the Commonwealth Fund, calls attention to another big problem that is still under the radar in the aftermath of the recent GOP tax bill. As he observes:

> *Fewer insured Americans and less-adequate public programs will mean fewer doctor visits, hospital stays, and drugs and devices sold. These cutbacks will ricochet through the economy, just like cutbacks in defense or infrastructure spending. Health care companies will employ fewer workers, who will buy fewer cars, homes, refrigerators, and vacations. Many will also lose health insurance. From a health care standpoint, the new tax bill is all about de-stimulus.* [26]

Concluding comment

State-based Medicaid will be a disaster for patients, and will be just a handout to private insurers as they get out from under the ACA's requirements. We can anticipate an even less efficient system than we now have and a whole new round of privatization and profiteering at the expense of patients and their families. That leads us to the next chapter.

References:

1. Jost, T. Universal access and delegation to states: Examining two currents in ACA replacement plans. *Health Affairs Blog*, January 20, 2017.

2. Lawson, A. Trump's budget calls for $1.8 trillion in cuts to earned benefits. *Social Security Works*, February 12, 2018.

3. Editorial Board, Donald Trump's nasty budget. *New York Times*, February 12, 2018.

4. Jan, T, Dewey, C, Goldstein, A et al. Trump wants to overhaul America's safety net with giant cuts to housing, food stamps, and health care. *The Washington Post*, February 12, 2018.

5. Ross, C. Trump health official Seema Verma has a plan to slash Medicaid rolls. Here's how. *STAT*, October 26, 2017.

6. Armour, S. More states weigh insurance mandates. *Wall Street Journal*, February 5, 2018: A5.

7. Sheen, R. As Congress moves to remove individual mandate, states seek their own version. *ACA Times*. January 8, 2018.

8. Goldstein, A. Indiana wins permission to adopt Medicaid work requirements. *The Washington Post*, February 2, 2018.

9. Itkowitz, C. There's a Medicaid 'subsidy cliff' health care officials are worried about. *The Washington Post*, July 19, 2018.

10. Solomon, J. As quoted by Galewitz, P, Bartolone, P. Trump's work-for-Medicaid rule puts work on states' shoulders. *Kaiser Health News*, January 12, 2018.

11. Alker, J. As quoted by Groppe, M. More than half of Indiana's alternative Medicaid recipients didn't make payment required for top service. *IndyStar*, May 8, 2017.

12. Pear, R. New health secretary faces first test as Idaho skirts federal law. *New York Times*, February 15, 2018.

13. Armour, S. Republicans try a patch for ACA. *Wall Street Journal*, February 16, 2017.

14. Appleby, J. Idaho Blue Cross jumps into controversial market for plans that bypass ACA rules. *Kaiser Health News*, February 14, 2018.

15. Lighty, M. New Medicaid work requirements will deny more care. *Sanders Institute*, November 15, 2017.

16. Sanger-Katz, M. The G.O.P. bill forces states to build health systems from scratch. That's hard. *New York Times*, September 21, 2017.

17. Cunningham, PW. PowerPost. The Health 202. Here are the most interesting things the new DHHS secretary said this week. *The Washington Post*, February 16, 2018**.**

18. Ibid # 15.

19. Editorial Board. Graham-Cassidy is another cynical effort that would deny health insurance to millions: Our view. *USA TODAY*, September 20, 2017.

20. Perreira, KM, Jones, DK. Oberlander, J. Reduce Medicaid spending? Look at Puerto Rico. *American Journal of Public Health*, December, 2017.

21. Sommers, BD, Naylor, D. Medicaid block grants and federalism: Lessons from Canada. *JAMA*, April 25, 2017.

22. Galewitz, P. Evaluation of Medicaid experiments by states, CMS are weak, GAO says. *Kaiser Health News*, February 23, 2018.

23. Artiga, S, Ubri, P, Zur, J. The effects of premiums and cost sharing on low-income populations. *Kaiser Family Foundation*, June 1, 2017.

24. Hellman, J. Study: Medicaid block grants would save feds $150 billion. *The Hill*, February 6, 2017.

25. Ross, C. In states that didn't expand Medicaid, hospital closures have spiked. STAT, January 8, 2018.

26. Blumenthal, D. How the new U. S. tax plan will affect health care. *Harvard Business Review*, December 19, 2017.

CHAPTER 5

INCREASING PRIVATIZATION
OF HEALTH CARE

Trump's signature brand of wheeling and dealing fits neatly in the recent tradition of running government "like a business." For decades, the corporate world has increasingly become the exemplar of good governance, and the market has come to stand for economic efficiency. These claims have fed into a trend of creeping privatization, which has weakened democratic public control over public goods, expanded corporate power, and widened economic and political inequality. Some of this trend has been driven by the desire to save public funds, and some of it by pure ideology.

—Jeremy Mohler and Donald Cohen [1]

The above observation cuts to the heart of ongoing trends in privatizing health care, based on a long-standing myth, now a meme, that somehow the private sector is more efficient and provides more value than the public sector. This has been disproven in our country over many decades, and privatization continues to be detrimental to the public interest.

This chapter has three goals: (1) to briefly bring some historical perspective to this claim, which should have been abandoned years ago in health care; (2) to describe the extent and results of privatization of U. S. health care; and (3) to compare private vs. social health insurance in terms of the extent to which they serve the public interest.

Brief Historical Perspective to Privatizing Health Care

Medicare was the first public program to be privatized, aided especially by passage by Congress of the Tax Equity and Fiscal Responsibility Act (TEFRA) in 1982. That bill allowed Medicare to contract with HMOs and pay them 95 percent of what traditional Medicare would pay for fee-for-service (FFS) care in beneficiaries' county of residence. The claim at the time was that private was more efficient and less expensive, but this was just a "bait and switch" gambit. A gaming system was soon launched by which privatized Medicare would pay *much more* than for traditional Medicare. By 1989, a report by Mathematica Policy Research, under contract to the Health Care Financing Administration (HCFA), found that Medicare was paying 15-33 percent more to private Medicare HMOs than for FFS care in traditional Medicare. [2] Overpayments reached about $283 *billion* between 1985 and 2008. [3]

Privatized Medicare received a big boost with the 1994 elections, when Republicans took control of both the House and Senate for the first time since 1954. Disregarding all experience with the grossly inflated costs of private Medicare programs, House Speaker Newt Gingrich, as part of the GOP's Contract with America, set out to hand over Medicare as a federal "entitlement program" to the private sector. In his famous words:

> *If we can solve Medicare, I think we will govern for a generation.* [4]

Here are three ways which show that the private sector in an unfettered health care marketplace fails to serve patients' best interests:

- According to a 2004 report, a nine-year tracking study of 12 major health care markets found these four barriers to efficiency of markets: (1) providers' market power; (2) absence of potentially efficient provider systems; (3) employers' inability to push the system toward efficiency and quality; and (4) insufficient competition among health plans. [5]
- Corporatization and consolidation have increased in recent years throughout the medical-industrial complex, including among insurers, hospital systems, nursing homes, the drug industry, and dialysis centers. As their market shares grow, they have more latitude to set prices to what the traffic will bear.
- Responding to their shareholders, corporate stakeholders pursue the business "ethic" seeking maximal revenue well beyond the service tradition.

Almost one-third of Medicare's 55 million beneficiaries are now in private Medicare plans, as well as more than one-half of 66 million people enrolled in Medicaid. [6] Today, House Speaker Paul Ryan is singing the same song as Gingrich in an effort to further privatize and cut federal responsibility for Medicare and Medicaid as "entitlement programs" in an effort to reduce the growing federal deficit resulting from the recently passed GOP tax plan.

Joseph Stiglitz, Nobel Laureate in Economics and former chief economist at the World Bank, has noted the clash between markets and social justice in this way:

Markets do not lead to efficient outcomes, let alone outcomes that comport with social justice. As a result, there is often good reason for government intervention to improve the efficiency of the market. Just as the Great Depression should have made it evident that the market often does not work as well as its advocates claim, our recent Roaring Nineties should have made it self-evident that the pursuit of self-interest does not necessarily lead to overall economic efficiency. [7]

Privatization Across U. S. Health Care

Time after time, whatever part of our health care system we look at, we find that privatization brings higher costs, less efficiency, less service, more bureaucracy, profiteering and often corruption. Privatized companies and contractors keep coming back to the public till and taxpayers for more money as their inefficiencies mount, in every case disproving their claimed efficiencies. Figure 5.1 shows the extent of for-profit ownership of health care providers across our health care system as of 2016.

Figure 5.1

EXTENT OF FOR-PROFIT OWNERSHIP, 2016

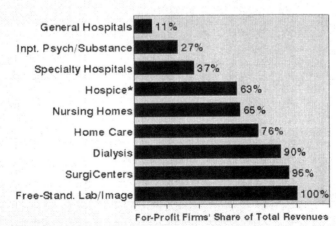

For-Profit Firms' Share of Total Revenues

Source: Commerce Dept. Service Annual Surveys and MedPac. Data are Q1, 2016 or most recent available. *Data are for share of establishments.

Let's take a look at how the private sector performs in five major areas of our health care system, with a view to how they serve their own self-interest vs. the public interest.

1. Medicare

The experience of privatized Medicare is a poster child for the abuses of corporate promises. The federal government has been very friendly to privatized Medicare in so many ways, including overpayments compared to traditional Medicare. The original idea that private Medicare plans would receive just 95 percent of FFS Medicare fell by the wayside early on.

Figure 5.2 shows that overpayments to private Medicare plans reached $173.7 billion between 2008 and 2016, despite any attempts by the ACA to rein them in. [8] All of these overpayments can be traced to up-coding and other ways used by private insurers to inflate the severity of their enrollees' conditions. Compared to traditional Medicare, privatized Medicare plans have consistently been more expensive, less efficient, less reliable, more restrictive in choice of physician and hospital, and have administrative costs about five times higher. [9] Ongoing lobbying by corporate stakeholders have led Congress to turn a blind eye to these overpayments.

Private Medicare plans game the system to avoid sicker, more costly enrollees, many of whom are dis-enrolled as their access is cut to preferred physicians, hospitals, and necessary drug treatment. A recent article by Sam Baker in *Axios Vitals* describes the startup of a new private Medicare insurer, Devoted Health, which has already raised $62 million and will start in 2019. Former DHHS Secretary Kathleen Sibelius is on its Board, as is former Senate Majority Leader Bill Frist. As Baker observes:

Medicare Advantage is where the big money is. The ACA marketplaces grab a lot of headlines, but they are a blip on the radar when compared with the hundreds of billions of dollars tied up in private Medicare plans and care for seniors. [10]

Figure 5.2

MEDICARE OVERPAYS PRIVATE PLANS

Total Overpayments 2008-2016: $173.7.billion

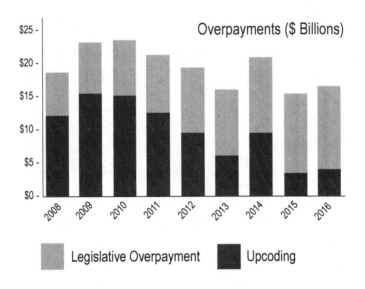

2. Medicaid

Privatized Medicaid follows the same pattern as for privatized Medicare. One such example is Tennessee Medicaid plans, operated by Blue Cross BlueShield of Tennessee, UnitedHealthcare, and Anthem, with their inadequate physician networks, long waits for care, and denials of many treatments, even as these insurers take away more profits. [11] A 2016 report by auditors at DHHS's Office of Inspector General estimated that Florida paid about $26 million over five years for coverage of people who had already died, mostly as a result of outdated information on state databases and a lack of collaboration among different agencies. [12]

3. Veterans Administration

After failing to fully repeal the ACA, deep-pocketed conservatives, driven by Koch money, have turned their sights on privatizing the VA, again falsely claiming that private would be more efficient. After 16 years of war, the already underfunded VA has been attacked for its long waiting times as the numbers of returning veterans with major medical and mental health problems increased their workloads. A battle has emerged between the majority of veterans and such long-standing organizations as Veterans of Foreign Wars and the American Legion and a new pro-privatization group, Concerned Veterans of America. [13]

The VA cares for almost 9 million veterans each year and has been more effective than private plans in improving quality of care, containing costs, and implementing electronic medical records. Table 5.1 shows how the quality of care in VA hospitals compares with non-VA hospitals, based on studies by RAND and the Agency for Healthcare Research and Quality (AHRQ). [14]

As well-funded conservative lobbyists press their case for privatizing the VA to congressional Republicans and the Trump administration, the Trump budget for the VA is 6 percent larger than last year's but one-third of the budget goes to private sector VA care, with only 1.3 percent to the VA itself. According to a 2017 wait time survey by Merritt Hawkins, wait times in the private sector, averaging about 24 days, are not much better than at a VA facility. Multiple polls have shown that a majority of veterans are satisfied with VA care and would rather see increased VA funding than money being funneled to the private sector. Will Fischer, a Marine Corp veteran who deployed to Iraq in 2004, brings us this insight:

> By making [private-sector care programs] mandatory, [VA officials] will be then pulling money out of other VA programs to fulfill the obligation of [private-sector programs] being mandatory—thus turning the VA into a slush fund for hospital executives and private care. [15]

TABLE 5.1

QUALITY OF CARE IN VA VERSUS NON-VA HOSPITALS

Health Indicator	VA Score*	National Sample**
Overall	67%	51%
Chronic care	72%	59%
Lung disease	69%	59%
Heart disease	73%	70%
Depression	80%	62%
Diabetes	70%	47%
Hypertension	78%	65%
High cholesterol	64%	53%
Osteoarthritis	65%	57%
Preventive care	64%	44%
Acute care	53%	55%
Screening	68%	46%
Diagnosis	73%	61%
Treatment	56%	41%
Follow-up	73%	58%

* 596 VA patients ** 992 patients at non-VA hospitals
Data: RandCorp; Agency for Healthcare Research & Quality

Source: Arnst, C. The best medical care in the U.S. *Business Week*, July 17, 2006

4. Mental Health Care

We've had a long-term system problem in this country due to lack of parity of coverage between mental health and substance abuse problems and medical/surgical conditions. This situation led to passage by Congress of the Mental Health Parity and Addiction Act of 2008 (MHPAAA). The intent of that law was to prevent group health plans from imposing less favorable limitations on those benefits than on medical/surgical benefits. Despite that legislation, this problem is ongoing. Milliman Inc., a national risk management and health care consulting company, in a study covering all 50 states and the District of Columbia, found that in 2015:

- Behavioral care was 4 to 6 times more likely to be covered by insurers *out-of-network* than for medical and surgical care.
- Insurers pay primary care providers 20 percent more for the same types of care as they pay mental health and addiction specialists.
- There is wide variation from one state to another; in New Jersey, 45 percent of office visits for behavioral health care were out-of-network.
- As a result, because of the high proportion of out-of-network behavioral care, these patients are more likely to face high out-of-pocket costs, even with insurance, which for many are unaffordable. [16]

Partly because of insurers' reimbursement policies, there is a critical shortage of mental health and substance abuse professionals. Narrow behavioral health networks typically do not have enough therapists available.

To make matters worse, separately and without explanation, the Trump administration has recently frozen the National Registry of Evidence-based Programs and Practices (NREPP), which was launched in 1997 to help find effective interventions for preventing and treating mental illness and substance abuse disorders. [17]

There is another enormous problem that makes the care of mental illness and substance abuse disorders even more challenging—the under-recognized growth of privatized prisons. This trend started in the 1980s, and by 2008 private prisons were big business with about 18 corporations guarding 10,000 prisoners in 27 states. At that time, 16 percent of the nation's 2 million prisoners were mentally ill, and would receive no treatment in prison. Wall Street investors have been happy with the profits that were possible by having the inmates work for as little as 17 cents per hour, or $20 per month for work up to 6 hours a day. The profit potential is further increased because so many people are being jailed for non-violent crimes, with long prison sentences for possession of microscopic quantities of illegal drugs, as well as passage of laws in some states that require minimum sentencing regardless of the circumstances. [18]

Today, in 2018, for-profit private prisons are a $5 billion industry that controls about 126,000 lives. They operate 65 percent of the country's detention beds. It is mostly opaque and almost entirely unaccountable. [20] Still another big problem is that private prisons prey on the poor and mentally ill, whereby poverty is criminalized by a mass incarceration system. The U. S. has more people in jail that anywhere else on the planet. Moreover, there is what turns out to be a loan shark operation to jail the poor for fines and bail. People are arrested on minor matters, held in jail on bail for $500, $1,000 or much more, have to plead guilty when that is unaffordable, then squeezed by a payment plan. It is estimated that 10 million people nationally owe some $50 billion in court debt. [20]

5. EMS services

In the wake of the 2008-2009 recession, many cities and towns across the country struggled to afford ambulance services. Private equity stepped in as new private ambulance companies sprouted up with a mission to make as much money as possible from what should be a public service. A 2016 report from the *New York Times* exposed their bad practices that often endangered the lives of patients. As they cut costs, raised prices, and adopted aggressive billing practices, ambulances often had expired medications, problems with life-saving equipment, regular breakdowns, delayed response times, even with no ambulances available on some occasions. "E. R. shopping" was a common practice whereby ambulances raided E. R.s for supplies. [21]

The Ongoing Debate over Private vs. Social Health Insurance

In its 1999 report, Medicare and the American Social Contract, a study panel of the National Academy of Social Insurance (NASI), noted these three key findings:

- Medicare was created as a response to a serious problem: The private market did not and could not work for a large population of the nation's elderly and disabled population.
- Medicare was originally designed as a social insurance program, rather than a social welfare program.
- Decisions about Medicare's future, including its ability to deal with health care utilization and costs, will not (and cannot) be made on purely economic or medical criteria.

Instead, seven criteria were recommended to be considered and weighed against each other as values and public concerns in the ongoing debate over Medicare's future: financial security, equity, efficiency, affordability over time, political accountability, political sustainability, and maximizing individual liberty. [22]

Traditional fee-for-service (FFS) Medicare has held fast to
these criteria in providing universal coverage to seniors and disabled
enrollees, and has consistently performed much better than privatized
Medicare across the board, as shown by Table 5.2. [23]

TABLE 5.2

CAMPARATIVE FEATURES OF PRIVATIZED AND PUBLIC MEDICARE

PRIVATIZED MEDICARE	ORIGINAL MEDICARE
Experience-rated eligibility	Universal coverage
Managed competition	Social insurance as earned right
Defined contribution	Defined benefits
Segmented risk pool	Broad risk pool
Market pricing to risk	Administered prices
More volatile access & benefits	More reliable access & benefits
Increased cost sharing	Less cost sharing
Less accountability	Potential for more accountability
Less choice of provider & hospital	Full choice of provider & hospital
Less well distributed	Well distributed
Less efficiency, higher overhead	More efficiency, lower overhead

Source: Geyman, JP. *Shredding the Social Contract The Privatization of Medicare.*
Monroe, ME. *Common Courage Press*, 2006, p.206

With increasing privatization of public plans in a market-based
health care economy, we see higher costs, less efficiency, more
bureaucracy and less accountability compared to public programs.
Continuing with Medicare as an example of this pattern, the 2017
Commonwealth Fund International Health Policy Survey of Older
Adults in eleven countries found that "the U. S. elderly face a 'triple

whammy' as they experience higher cost sharing, higher levels of economic vulnerability, and dramatically higher health care costs—with prescription drugs often two or three times as expensive in the United States as in the other countries studied. [24]

In their 2014 book, *Social Insurance: America's Neglected Heritage and Contested Future*, Theodore Marmor, Jerry Mashaw and John Pakutka draw this important conclusion about the need for more government involvement to counteract the adverse effects of "free market" policies in our health care:

> *In health care, the "invisible hand" [of the free market] fails to drive down costs, improve quality, or ensure distributional outcomes that are regarded as fair. We can tinker with the rules, regulations and payment schemes that govern medical care, but the forces that increase the demands for and supply of more care are relentless. Only powerful countervailing institutions can keep them under control. Only governments have the necessary authority, assuming they have the political will to use it.* [25]

Concluding comment:

We are seeing ongoing corporate welfare in the medical-industrial complex, as in so many other parts of our economy. Because of the economic and political power of the private health insurance industry, we have yet to deal with the obvious advantages of universal coverage as can be provided under a system of not-for-profit social insurance, as we will discuss in Chapter 16. For now, let's look in the next chapter at how patient protections, as provided under the ACA, have been lost under the onslaught of Trump sabotage.

References:

1.   Mohler, J, Cohen, D. The incoming privatization assault. *The American Prospect*, April 24, 2017, p. 97.

2.   General Accounting Office (GAO). Medicare: Reasonableness of Health Maintenance Organizations Not Assured. GAO/HRD-89-41. Washington D.C.: Government Printing Office, 1989.

3.   Trivedi, AN, Gribla, RC, Jiang, L et al. Duplicate federal payments to dual enrollees in Medicare Advantage plans and the Veterans Administration Health Care System. *JAMA* 308 (1): 67-72, 2012.

4.   Smith, DG. *Entitlement Politics: Medicare and Medicaid 1995-2001*. New York. *Aldine de Gruyter*, 2002: 71, citing Congressional Quarterly Almanac, 1995, p. 73.

5.   Nichols, LM et al. Are market forces strong enough to deliver efficient health care systems? Confidence is waning. *Health Affairs* (*Millwood*) 23 (2): 8-21, 2004.

6.   Pear, R. As Medicare and Medicaid turn 50, use of private health plans surges. *New York Times*, July 30, 2015: A 12.

7.   Stiglitz, JE. Evaluating economic change. *Daedalus* 133/3, Summer, 2004.

8.   Geruso, M, Layton, T. Upcoding inflates Medicare costs in excess of $2 billion annually. *UT News*, University of Texas at Austin, June 18, 2015.

9.   Healthcare-NOW! Single-Payer Activist Guide to the Affordable Care Act. Philadelphia, PA, 2013, p. 22.

10. Baker, S. The newest Medicare startup. *Axios Vitals*, October 24, 2017.

11. Himmelstein, DU, Woolhandler, S. The post-launch problem: The Affordable Care Act's persistently high administrative costs. *Health Affairs Blog*, May 27, 2017.

12. Chang, D. Florida paid Medicaid insurers $26 million to cover dead people, report says. *Miami Herald*, December 13, 2016.

13. Kesling, B. Kochs to push to reshape VA services. *Wall Street Journal*, November 4-5, 2017.

14. Arnst, C. The best medical care in the U. S. *Business Week*, July 17, 2006.

15. Fischer, W. As quoted by Bernd, C. How the Koch-backed effort to privatize the Veterans Health Administration jeopardizes everyone's health care future. *Truthout*, July 2, 2017.

16. Gold, J. If your insurer covers few therapists, is that really mental health parity? *Kaiser Health News*, November 30, 2017.

17. Sun, LH, Eiperin, J. Trump administration freezes database of addiction and mental health programs. *The Washington Post*, January 10, 2018.

18. Pelaez, V. The prison industry in the United States: Big business or a new form of slavery? *Global Research*, January 25, 2018.

19. Eisen, LB. Private prisons lock up thousands of Americans with almost no oversight. *Time*, November 8, 2017.

20. Karlin, M. Jailing the poor for fines and bail is a government-operated loan shark operation. *Truthout*, February 4, 2018.

21. Ivory, D, Protess, B, Daniel, J. When you dial 911 and Wall Street answers, *New York Times*, June 25, 2016.

22. National Academy of Social Insurance, *Medicare and the American Social Contract*, February 1999.

23. Geyman, JP. *Shredding the Social Contract: The Privatization of Medicare.* Monroe, ME. *Common Courage Press*, 2006, p. 206.

24. Osborn, R, Doty, MM, Moulds, D et al. Older Americans were sicker and faced more financial barriers to health care than their counterparts in other countries. *Health Affairs*, November 15, 2017.

25. Marmor, TR, Mashaw, JL, Pakutka, J. *Social Insurance: America's Neglected Heritage and Contested Future.* Los Angeles, CA. *Sage Copress*, 2014, p. 128.

CHAPTER 6

LOSS OF PATIENT PROTECTIONS

Well, we are protecting pre-existing conditions. [The GOP health care bills in Congress in 2017] will be as good on pre-existing conditions as Obamacare.

—President Donald Trump [1]

Another outright lie by Trump, talking about GOP bills in Congress in May 2017, which would have eliminated many of the patient protections of the ACA. We saw in the last two chapters the various ways by which the ACA has been sabotaged, together with shifting responsibility from the federal government to the states. These actions will remove protections assured by the ACA, such as its banning of health insurance rates based on preexisting conditions, coverage of essential health benefits without annual lifetime limits, and guaranteed renewability.

This chapter has two goals: (1) to describe the kinds of losses of patient protections as a result of Trump's executive orders and recent administrative policies of Department of Health and Human Services (DHHS); and (2) to discuss the impacts on patients of the loss of these protections.

Loss of Patient Protections

As enacted in 2010, the ACA established that: "All marketplace plans must cover treatment for pre-existing medical conditions. No insurance plan can reject you, charge you more, or refuse to pay for essential health benefits for any condition you had before your coverage started. Once you're enrolled, the plan can't deny you coverage or raise your rates based only on your health."

These are some of the many ways that the Trump administration has withered away most of these consumer protections of plans offered on the ACA's exchanges:

1. *Pre-existing conditions.*

Under state waivers that will be passed out readily by DHHS under the Trump administration, insurers will be free in many states to market plans that deny coverage for pre-existing conditions and/or to charge big hikes in premiums if coverage is offered. Common reasons for denial include such conditions as cancer, asthma, hepatitis, and depression. According to the Center for American Progress, premiums would increase by $4,340 for patients with asthma and by $28,660 a year for patients having breast cancer, thereby pricing many out of the marketplace. [2]

In 2015, the AARP estimated that about 40 percent of adults age 50 to 64 would have pre-existing conditions rendering their coverage difficult or impossible to get. Based in its study estimating how this problem would vary from one state to another before the ACA, Figure 6.1 gives us some idea as to how many people will be so affected across the country. [3] As Sabrina Corlette, research professor at Georgetown University's Health Policy Institute, observes:

The protection your insurance provides could depend a lot on where you live. In some states, over time, [patients with chronic illness] might find it increasingly difficult to find insurance companies that will offer plans that cover their needs.[4]

FIGURE 6.1

PERCENT OF ADULTS AGES 50-64 WITH A DECLINABLE PRE-EXISTING CONDITION, UNDER PRE-ACA MEDICAL UNDERWRITING PRACTICES, 2015

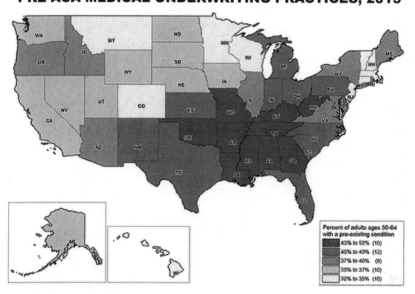

Source: AARP Public Policy Institute Analysis of data from the 2015 Behavioral Risk Factor Surveillance System (SRF55).

The new landscape of TrumpCare will not pass the Jimmy Kimmel test, which evolved in the aftermath of his newborn son, Billy, born with a heart defect that required surgery and very large bills. On his late-night show, he made a passionate plea that "no parent should ever have to decide if they can afford to save their child's life." He invited Senator Bill Cassidy (R-LA), sponsor of the failed Graham-Cassidy bill in 2017, to his show, where they discussed the newly termed "Jimmy Kimmel test" - "No family should be denied medical care, emergency or otherwise, because they can't afford it."

Though Sen. Cassidy seemed to agree with that notion on the show, his legislative effort would have failed to answer the affordability part, which in this instance could have reached lifetime cap territory.[5]

Dean Baker, senior economist at The Center for Economic and Policy Research, commenting on the Trump administration's latest attacks on the ACA:

> *To my view, the key part of Obamacare was creating a unified insurance market where anyone can get insurance regardless of their health and this is destroying that. So what this means is we'll be back to the world pre-Obamacare where, suppose you have a heart condition, suppose you are a cancer survivor, you either won't be able to get insurance at all or if you do have a company that's offering to sell you insurance, they're gonna want 50, 60, or 70,000 dollars a year . . . . not many people could afford to pay that.* [6]

2. *Increasing premiums*

Average ACA exchange market premiums increased by 28 percent from 2014 to 2017. [7] Premiums will go much higher with deletion of the individual mandate and as insurers charge seniors five times as much as younger enrollees, compared to the 3:1 ratio of the ACA. Coverage will go down with promulgation of short-term, limited-coverage plans and association health plans, and other means by which the Trump administration has opened the door for insurers to expand new markets with "junk insurance." Short-term plans are expected to attract many healthy, young people, thus further segmenting risk pools and raising premiums for older and sicker people.

Insurers had already factored in the loss of CSR payments as they raised premiums for 2018. The consulting firm Avalere Health projected that premiums would go up by 69 percent in Iowa, 65 percent in Wyoming, and 64 percent in Utah. [8] A recent estimate by the Urban Institute projected that premiums for 2019 will increase by 18.2 percent in 41 states plus the District of Columbia. [9] Kevin Lucia, research professor and project director at Georgetown University's Health Policy Institute, predicts:

> *If consumers think Obamacare premiums are high today, wait until people flood into these short-term and association health plans. The Trump administration will bring rates down substantially for healthy people, but woe unto those who get a condition and have to go back into Obamacare.* [10]

3. Essential health benefits excluded

As we saw in Chapter 3, there are various ways that insurers can avoid coverage of any of the ACA's ten essential health benefits, especially through short-term limited-benefit plans and association health plans marketed to employers that cross state lines. Coverage will vary greatly from one state to another, and enrollees can expect to pay much higher out-of-pocket costs for health care. Enrollees will have to look carefully at the fine print of their plans to see what exclusions are built into their policies, such as whether chemotherapy is covered for patients with cancer. Insurers will also be able to exit insufficiently profitable markets without concern for their enrollees.

4. New Medicaid restrictions

Some states are tightening their eligibility requirements, setting annual and/or lifetime caps (such as three to five years), and/or enforcing premiums with loss of coverage if not paid. Ten states have already applied for federal waivers to implement work requirements for their Medicaid recipients. Under TrumpCare, they will have these new ways to lose their coverage if they can't find work for various reasons—live in areas of persistent unemployment, got laid off during a recession, have seasonal jobs, or don't get enough work from their employer as they want. [11] Those who do not meet work requirements for Medicaid are unlikely to receive premium tax credits for plans offered on the ACA's exchanges, with many being unable to afford such coverage. [12] As Chad Bolt, senior policy manager at Indivisible, observes:

> *Work requirements don't help the unemployed or underemployed to find work. [It] just punishes them when they're down—which is exactly what the Trump administration wants to do.* [13]

In addition, implementing a work requirement policy for Medicaid adds a whole new layer of costly bureaucracy to the program.

Impacts of Lost Patient Protections

Based on the above attacks on the ACA's protections, these are the inevitable consequences of the GOP's sabotage of the law without any replacement plan of their own.

1. *Unaffordable premiums*

The most popular ACA plans will see premium increases by an average of 34 percent in 2018. Molina Healthcare, one of the largest marketplace insurers, will increase its premiums by an average of 55 percent. [14]

2. *Unaffordable care especially for older and sicker people*

Even if insured, people will find their cost sharing increased for less coverage. As a result, they will pay more for actual care, if they can afford it at all. The proposed rule by DHHS for short-term, limited-duration plans even acknowledges that this coverage is "exempt from the ACA's individual market requirements because it is *not* individual health insurance coverage." [15] Industry consultant Robert Laszewski predicts that we will have two different markets: a Wild West frontier called short-term medical . . . and a high-risk pool called Obamacare." [16]

3. *Impacts on Medicare*

The Trump budget released in February 2018 for fiscal year 2019 would cut the budget of Medicare by $554 billion. Private Medicare Advantage plans cover about one-third of the 55 million people on Medicare. Sicker patients will have to leave their plans as insurers cut access to preferred physicians, hospitals, and necessary drug treatment.

4. *Impacts on Medicaid*

The proposed Trump budget for Medicaid in fiscal year 2019 calls for a cut of $1.3 *trillion*. There are almost 25 million non-elderly adults enrolled in Medicaid. Although many gained coverage in the 32 states that expanded Medicaid under the ACA, most are still the usual population—children, people with disabilities, and non-elderly adults without Social Security. Nearly eight in ten of these Medicaid enrollees are in working families, and a majority are working themselves. Those who can't find work or are limited by disabilities will find themselves vulnerable to loss of coverage under TrumpCare's state waivers. [17]

5. *More restricted networks*

This will happen as insurers cut providers to maximize profits, leaving many patients having to pay big increases in costs of out-of-network care.

6. *Less choice*

Recall from the last chapter that there will soon be 454 counties with only one insurer (page 55) with a growing number of counties with none.

7. *Increased numbers of uninsured*

The CBO has projected that 13 million more people will be without health insurance by 2026, and this number is likely to be far higher as insurers in more states restrict their definition of essential health benefits. [18]

8. *Increased numbers of underinsured*

Given the new freedom of insurers to market very skinny plans, we can anticipate tens of millions of people to be underinsured, all more a problem given the lack of cost and price constraints under TrumpCare.

9. *Impacts on employer-sponsored insurance*

Under association health plans, small businesses can join associations, based on certain kinds of professional, trade or interest groups in order to offer insurance across state lines with minimal standards for coverage. This will be another step toward increasing the numbers of underinsured. [19]

10. *Impacts on women's health care*

These will be adverse as many insurers delete maternal health from their offerings. The GOP in many states has been cutting Planned Parenthood clinics and services, and that trend will likely continue. Already, the number of Planned Parenthood clinics across the country has been reduced from 860 to 600 in the last 13 years; prenatal services have been cut by more than two-thirds as the number of breast exams have been cut by almost one-half. [20]

11. *Further fracturing of the nation's safety net*

As responsibility for health care programs shifts to the states, we will see funding cuts to community health centers, hospitals, nursing homes and other safety net programs, including CHIP and SNAP (food stamps) because of lack of funds at the state level. Rural hospitals will be especially hard hit, with 83 closures already since 2010. [21]

Concluding comment

Alex Azar, Trump's pick to head DHSS and former drug company executive, was so proud of his proposed rule to expand short-term, limited-duration health insurance plans, that he took this kind of credit:

> *Americans need more choices in health insurance so they can find coverage that meets their needs. The status quo is failing too many Americans who face skyrocketing costs and fewer and fewer choices. The Trump administration is taking action so individuals and families have access to quality, affordable healthcare that works for them.* [22]

That boast is disingenuous and hypocritical, given that many millions of Americans will have far fewer choices for access to affordable health care, there is no cost containment in sight, and no attention has been paid as to how to define "affordable." We can conclude that this is just another lie from the Trump administration. Many millions of Americans will be worse off than ever before, and private health insurers will enjoy another giveaway from the government even as they find new ways to profiteer on the backs of many millions of Americans.

References:

1. Trump, DJ. As quoted by Robert Dhondrup, *Liar-in-Chief: The Lies of President Trump*. May 1, 2017.

2. Pitt, WR. Graham-Cassidy is evil incarnate. *Truthout*, September 24, 2017.

3. Bump, P. How many with preexisting conditions would be priced out of coverage under Cassidy-Graham? *The Washington Post*, September 21, 2017.

4. Hancock, J, Bluth, R. Promises made to protect preexisting conditions prove hollow. *Kaiser Health News*, June 22, 2017.

5. Yahr, E. Jimmy Kimmel gets heated about health-care bill, says Sen. Bill Cassidy 'lied right to my face.' *The Washington Post*, September 20, 2017.

6. Baker, D, as quoted by Wilpert, G. Will Trump's latest attack on Obamacare strike a death blow? *The Real News.com*, February 22, 2018.

7. The high cost of healthcare: Patients see greater cost-shifting and reduced coverage in exchange markets 2014-2017. Physicians for Fair Coverage. Research by Avalere, July 2018.

8. Milbank, D. Trump just told the truth. He may wish he hadn't. *The Washington Post*, December 20, 2017.

9. Hiltzik, M. The stupidity of TrumpCare: Government will spend $33 billion more to cover 8.9 million fewer Americans, as premiums soar. *Los Angeles Times*, February 26, 2018.

10. Lucia, K. As quoted by Appleby, J. Trump administration proposes rule to loosen curbs on short-term health plans. *Kaiser Health News*, February 20, 2018.

11. Rosenbaum, S, Wachino, V, Gunsalus, R et al. State 1115 proposals to reduce Medicaid eligibility: Assessing their scope and projected impact. *The Commonwealth Fund*, January 11, 2018.

12. Andrews, M. Refusing to work for Medicaid may not translate to subsidies for ACA plan. *Kaiser Health News*, February 27, 2018.

13. Bolt, C. Trump launches 'truly savage' attack on Medicaid by pushing work requirement. *Common Dreams*, January 11, 2018.

14. Mathews, AW. Molina to exit two exchanges. *Wall Street Journal*, August 3, 2017.

15. Azar, A. Trump administration works to give relief to Americans facing high premiums, fewer choices. U. S. Department of Health & Human Services, February 20, 2018.

16. Laszewski, R. As quoted by Appleby, J. Trump administration proposed rule to loosen curbs on short-term health plans. *Kaiser Health News*, February 20, 2018.

17. Garfield, R, Rudowitz, R, Damico, A. Understanding the intersection of Medicaid and work. *Kaiser Family Foundation*, January 5, 2018.

18. Ibid # 2.

19. Appleby, J. Association health plans: A favorite GOP approach to coverage poised for comeback. *Kaiser Health News*, October 6, 2017.

20. Firozi, PW. Planned Parenthood goes on the offensive. *The Washington Post*, February 14, 2018.

21. Ross, C. In states that didn't expand Medicaid, hospital closures have spiked. *STAT*, January 8, 2018.

22. Azar, A. Ibid # 15.

CHAPTER 7

DEREGULATION OF HEALTH CARE

A constant mantra during Trump's campaign and first year in office has been to claim that we are over-regulated and that somehow deregulation of health, safety, labor, financial, and environmental sectors will somehow get us on a better track in this country. His simplistic and non-coherent policy seems to be that regulations are bad, take away jobs, and deregulation will improve the economy. He issued an executive order ten days after taking office that government agencies should kill two rules for every new one they propose. His Cabinet has been loyal to this cause and have taken on the "deconstruction of the administrative state," as urged on by Steve Bannon, Trump's former policy guru. This direction toward small government has had the strong support of the Freedom Caucus (including House Tea Party members), many trade organizations (including the Chamber of Commerce and the National Association of Manufacturers), and corporate lobbyists. [1]

This chapter has two goals: (1) to describe the kinds of deregulatory actions that have been taken across various parts of the health care system; and (2) to ask and try to answer whether U. S. health care can be regulated in the public, not corporate interest?

Deregulation Across the Health Care System

Let's look at how the emphasis on deregulation in recent years, has accelerated during the Trump administration, and has played out in eight parts of our health care system.

Insurance industry

Regulation of private health insurance has always been lax. For many years, most regulatory authority has been given to the states, where the insurance lobby dominates state capitols. Insurance regulators in the states have long had a cozy relationship with industry. As one example, the Center for Public Integrity has found that one-half of state insurance commissioners who have left their jobs in the last ten years have gone to work for the industry they were supposedly regulating. [2]

The ACA continued that trend, with minimal federal oversight over states. Now there is even less federal oversight, with big variations from one state to another. As we have seen in earlier chapters, states now have even more leeway under TrumpCare. The DHHS permits marketing of plans that do not comply with the ACA's regulations, which require coverage of all ten essential health benefits, banning of annual and lifetime limits, and not setting premiums based on age, health status and history. Meanwhile, with little public scrutiny, private insurers are vacuuming up personal details of hundreds of Americans which can be used to raise premiums or deny coverage. [3]

Hospital industry

In contrast to the insurance industry, the hospital industry is over-regulated, but much of the regulatory process is fundamentally flawed. A recent report from the American Hospital Association describes the complexity and inefficiencies of this process. Health systems, hospitals, and post-acute providers, such as long-term care hospitals and skilled nursing facilities, must comply with 629 discrete regulatory requirements across nine domains. These requirements are promulgated by four different federal agencies, and are often duplicative. They must also comply with many stringent contract requirements imposed by payers, such as private Medicare and Medicaid plans and commercial payers. They spend $39 billion a year to meet these requirements. An average-size hospital employs 59 full-time people, more than one-quarter of whom are doctors and nurses, to stay in compliance. [4]

Despite this immense effort to comply with federal regulations, the burdensome process fails to meet the goal of best protecting the public. Most hospitals are accredited by a Joint Commission with a board mostly composed of executives of health systems it accredits as well as members named by health care lobbying groups. A national study of hospital inspection reports between 2014 and 2016 found that the vast majority of hospitals found to have safety violations kept their full 'Gold Seal of Approval.' [5] A 2016 study of 22 million hospital admissions concluded that patients are 3 times more likely to die in the worst hospitals and 13 times more likely to have medical complications compared to the best hospitals. [6]

Surgery centers

Surgery centers started almost 50 years ago as low-cost alternatives for minor surgical procedures. Since then their numbers have soared to more than 5,600 in the U. S., and they have become a hazard for many patients. A 2007 report by Medicare noted that "surgery centers have neither patient safety standards consistent with those in hospitals, nor are they required to have the trained staff and equipment needed to provide the breadth of intensity of care . . . Some procedures are unsafe to be handled at surgery centers." [7]

That far more regulation of surgery centers is needed is shown by these problems:

- Surgery centers take on many major surgical procedures, including complex spinal surgeries.
- More than 260 patients have died since 2013 after in-and-out care at U. S. surgery centers, many as a result of inadequate treatment of complications; it is not uncommon for staff to call 911 in these instances.
- At least 7,000 patients required transfer to a hospital in the year that ended in September 2017. [8]

Drug industry

The drug industry has effectively lobbied over many years to avoid price controls and other regulations over its promotion and marketing practices. Since 1993, it has managed a big effort through direct-to-consumer drug advertising, banned in many advanced countries, often with misinformation and false claims. The industry brought out a new argument in 2017 based on the First Amendment in an attempt to evade drug safety rules and sell more medications for off-label marketing of unapproved drugs. [9] The industry has long lobbied against importation of drugs from other countries and for faster action by the FDA for approvals with less rigorous oversight. Since 1962, the previous gold standard for FDA approval required "substantial evidence" of a drug's efficacy based on controlled clinical trials. The recent passage of the 21st Century Cures Act has drastically lowered the standards for FDA approval of new drugs to a new "standard" based on "real world evidence" (read non-rigorous uncontrolled observational data easily gamed by drug manufacturers through their marketing departments). [10]

The FDA itself is plagued by underfunding, lack of sufficient authority, and conflicts of interest. The industry supports much of the

FDA's budget through user fees. As the fox-in-the-henhouse, many reviewers on FDA panels have close ties to industry and one-half of all health care lobbyists are former government officials. [11]

Corporate greed trumps patient safety through this lax regulatory process. As just one of many examples, a study of FDA-approved drugs subsequently withdrawn from the market between 1993 and 2010 found that unsafe drugs were prescribed more than 100 million times in the U. S. before being recalled from the market. [12]

Medical device industry

The medical device industry is larger than most of us might think, with an enormous market ranging from cardiac pacemakers and defibrillators to lasers, hip and knee replacements. Also regulated by the FDA, this industry follows the same pattern as the drug industry, putting profits ahead of patient safety. A 2014 study reported in *JAMA Internal Medicine* found that 42 of 50 selected medical devices cleared by the FDA over five years lacked publicly available scientific evidence verifying their safety and effectiveness despite a 1990 law requiring such evidence. [13] Medical device manufacturers often delay notification to the FDA about negative experiences with their products, continue marketing them beyond adverse reports, and seek support from willing legislators. Johnson & Johnson's defective all-metal ASR hip replacement is one example of this delaying action, which ended up in the filing of some 5,000 lawsuits against the company. [14]

Nursing homes

Nursing homes have never been regulated in the public interest. Two-thirds of them are for-profit, placing profits ahead of service. Compared to not-for-profit nursing homes, for-profit chains are typically investor owned, have lower staffing levels, worse quality of care, and higher death rates. A report by the Inspector General in 2012 found that for-profit nursing homes overbilled Medicare by $1.5 billion a year for treatments that patients didn't need and never received. [15] Life Care Centers of America Inc., one of the nation's largest chains, settled the largest claim yet of $145 million with the federal government in 2016 for violations of the False Claims Act for having provided unreasonable and unnecessary therapy to many patients. [16]

The situation is now even worse under the Trump administration, which has rolled back many of the previous regulations on nursing homes. In February 2018, the administration imposed an 18-month moratorium on imposing fines or denials of federal payments when nursing homes fail to meet certain requirements, such as ensuring that they have adequate staffing or are using psychotropic drugs correctly. In opposition to this moratorium, a group of Democratic senators, led by Sen. Richard Blumenthal (D-CT) and Sen. Amy Klobuchar (D-MN), sent a letter to Alex Azar at DHHS, voicing serious concern that "this will inevitably weaken the safety of our nation's nursing homes and put patients, many of whom are elderly and wholly reliant on this care, at greater risk." [17]

Hospices

There is also inadequate regulation of hospices, two-thirds of which are for-profit. Compared to their not-for profit counterparts, for-profits offer fewer services and provide worse quality of care.[18] The number of for-profit hospices almost doubled from 2000 to 2013, with Medicare spending for that care going up by five-fold. A report from *The Washington Post* found the industry riddled with fraud and abuse, such as seeking out less sick patients who need less care and live longer and offering their employees to recruit patients. [19]

Laboratory tests

There is a large under recognized multi-billion-dollar-a-year business in "lab-developed tests" that is virtually unregulated. These tests have rarely been scrutinized by the FDA, gone through clinical trials, or been proven accurate or medically useful before going to market. As the adverse impacts of inaccurate tests have become widespread, the FDA is now trying to better regulate this industry, seeing these tests as the Wild West of medicine. Examples of tests with unproven effectiveness include the BRCA gene test for breast cancer, which has led some women to undergo bilateral mastectomies unnecessarily, and a KIF6 gene test as a way to detect a predisposition to heart disease. A study of 55 cancer-care and testing websites by researchers at Harvard and the Dana-Farber Cancer Center concluded that "most of the websites have little or no evidence substantiating the ability to improve patient outcome." [20]

Can Health Care Be Regulated in the Public Interest?

As is obvious from the foregoing, we have a poor track record in this country in trying to regulate the health care industry in the public interest. The regulatory process is lax or far too complex, ineffective, and hijacked by corporate stakeholders protecting their prerogatives in a free wheeling market-based system. Health care is being treated as just another commodity for sale on an open market that is oriented to increasing corporate revenues at the expense of patient care. This failure over many years leads us to question how and whether we can achieve regulatory protection of patient safety.

The idea that markets will self-correct has been proven wrong over many years. This situation is all the more challenging because of GOP control of Congress and the Trump administration, ideologically opposed as they are to more regulation and in favor of smaller government. The Trump administration has launched a deregulatory bonanza. As one example, penalties for corporate crime and misconduct of the country's 100 most profitable corporations dropped from about $17 billion a year during the Obama administration to just $1.1 billion in Trump's first year in office. [21]

It has become apparent that a larger role of government will be required if we are to achieve significant correction of unethical and profit-driven practices within the medical-industrial complex that put patients at risk. We need to come to grips with the concept that the goal of our health care should be to best advance the interests of patients, not corporate earnings, as so many other advanced countries around the world have done for years. The concept of the common good should be at the heart of health policy, which can never happen within the present culture of health care. As John Adams, the second president of the United States and one of our founding fathers, said:

Government is instituted for the common good: for the protection, safety, prosperity and happiness of the people; and not for the profit, honor, or private interest of any one man, family, or class of men.

The ACA introduced new supposedly "value-based" initiatives that theoretically might improve the quality of patient care, such as pay-for-performance" (P4P) report cards for physicians and accountable care organizations. Although we now have some 150 quality metrics in use for evaluating outpatient services, there is still no evidence that any of them improve care. Instead, aided by electronic health records that have largely become billing instruments, they consume much of physicians' and their staffs' time and are easily gamed by up-coding for maximal revenue, usually to physicians' employers. [22]

We know that up to one-third of all health care services provided are inappropriate, unnecessary, and even dangerous to patients in some instances. [23] But they are the result of a system based on maximal profits, not the best interests of patients.

In order to rein in the excesses of today's profit-driven health care system, we will need financing reform. The regulatory burden now being placed on health systems, hospitals, and post-acute care providers that require regular reporting across nine domains, leads Dr. Don McCanne, senior health policy fellow and past president of Physicians for a National Health Program, to say:

A quick look at the nine domains of regulatory overload is all you need to be reminded of the nightmare created by these evolving requirements. Inefficiencies, wasted resources, and provider burnout ensue, which negatively impact the primary mission of the health care system: patient care. . . . Think of the recoverable administrative waste that characterizes our fragmented health care financing system—most of which is in the private sector. We spend over a trillion dollars a year on administration, and somewhere around $300 billion to $500 billion is recoverable merely by transitioning to a well-designed single payer system. [24]

Concluding comment

Given that TrumpCare involves far less regulation than will be required to protect patients, it is time to move on to the next six chapters where we will describe the various ways that TrumpCare is failing, but also open up new opportunities to reform U. S. health care in the public interest.

References:

1. Steinzor, R. The war on regulation. *The American Prospect*, Spring 2017, pp. 72-76.
2. Mishak, MJ. Drinks, junkets and jobs. How the insurance industry courts state commissioners. *The Washington Post*, October 2, 2016.
3. Allen, M. Health insurers are vacuuming up details about you—and it may raise your rates. *ProPublica*, July 17, 2018.
4. Regulatory overload: Assessing the regulatory burden on health systems, hospitals, and post-acute care providers. *American Hospital Association*, October 2017.
5. Armour, S. Hospitals keep 'gold seal' despite woes. *Wall Street Journal*, September 9-10: A1, 2017.
6. Abelson, R. Go to the wrong hospital and you're 3 times more likely to die. *New York Times*, December 4, 2016.
7. Jewett, C, Alesia, M. Surgery centers boom, patients are paying with their lives. *Kaiser Health News* and *USA TODAY* Network, March 2, 2018.
8. Ibid # 7.
9. Feng, R. PhRMA's latest excuse for off-label marketing won't fly. *Public Citizen* 37 (1): Jan/Feb 2017, p. 1.
10. Gaffney, A. Congress just quietly handed drug companies a dangerous victory. *New Republic*, December 14, 2016.
11. Demko, P. Healthcare's hired hands: When the stakes rise in Washington, healthcare interests seek well-connected lobbying firms. *Modern Healthcare*, October 6, 2014.
12. Saluja, S, Woolhandler, S, Himmelstein, DU et al. Unsafe drugs were prescribed more than one hundred million times in the United States before being recalled. *Intl J Health Services*, June 14, 2016.
13. Burton, TM. FDA faulted over medical devices. *Wall Street Journal*, September 30, 2014.
14. Meier, B. Hip implants U. S. rejected sold overseas. *New York Times*, February 12, 2012: A1.
15. Waldman, P. For-profit nursing homes lead in overcharging while care suffers. *Bloomberg Business*, December 31, 2012.
16. Press release. Department of Justice, October 24, 2016.
17. Weixel, N. Dems seek reversal of nursing home regulatory rollback. *The Hill*, February 20, 2018.
18. Perry, J, Stone, R. In the business of dying: Questioning the commercialization of hospice. *J Law, Medicine, and Ethics*, May 18, 2011.

19. McCauley, L. Investigation reveals rampant fraud by privatized hospice groups. *Common Dreams*, December 17, 2013.

20. Burton, TM. The 'wild west' of medicine. *Wall Street Journal*, December 11, 2015: A1.

21. Johnson, J. Tracking tool shows fines for corporate misconduct have plummeted under Trump. *Common Dreams*, February 13, 2018.

22. Casalino, LP, Gans, , Weber, R et al. U. S. physician practices spend more than $15.4 billion annually to report quality measures. *Health Affairs*, March 2016.

23. Wenner, JB, Fisher, ES, Skinner, JS. Geography and the debate over Medicare reform. *Health Affairs Web Exclusive* W-103, February 13, 2001.

24. McCanne, D. Comment on Ibid # 4. The cost of regulatory overload. Quote of the Day, October 27, 2017.

How TrumpCare Is Failing

CHAPTER 8

DECLINING ACCESS TO AFFORDABLE HEALTH CARE

Health care is a social good, not a commodity, just like primary education, fire and police protection, and clean water. A market-based system is not only wasteful, it's immoral.

—Dr. Marcia Angell, former editor-in chief
of the *New England Journal of Medicine* [1]

This chapter, the first among six, will describe the various ways by which TrumpCare is certain to fail to meet the needs of Americans for affordable, quality health care.

Republicans are correct that the ACA left many needs unfulfilled, despite its success in bringing significant improvement to many millions of Americans. But everything Republicans have done to unravel the ACA, mostly by administrative means of the Trump administration, has made the situation far worse with no hope for improvement in sight. Trump's promises are hollow, disingenuous, and blatantly dishonest in touting what TrumpCare can do for us.

This chapter has two goals: (1) to describe eight different ways in which TrumpCare puts access to affordable care out of reach for much of the middle class as well as lower-income people; and (2) to briefly discuss how increasing inequality in American society further contributes to inadequate access to health care.

The Many Barriers to Access to Affordable Health Care

1. The uninsured

Despite progress under the ACA, there are now 28 million people without health insurance, almost 9 percent of the U. S. population. The uninsured include 6.3 percent of non-Hispanic whites, 10.5 percent of blacks, 16.0 percent of Latinos, 7.6 percent of Asians, and almost 20 percent of Native Americans. An additional 18 million non-elderly adults have a gap in coverage at some point during the year, according to the U. S. Census Bureau and the Commonwealth Fund. [2, 3] The most recent information on the uninsured rate, based on a third-quarter 2017 Gallup survey, puts the number of uninsured even higher at 12.3 percent of the population. [4]

Here is one example of what these abstract numbers mean to real people, which would be understandable in a third world country but not in this country with all its abundance.

> *Sarai was 25 years old when she died of Wilson's disease, an inherited disorder that leads to liver failure. She could have been cured by having a liver transplant, but was uninsured and was denied at two prominent liver transplant hospitals in Chicago for lack of coverage. Her physician signed her death certificate as liver failure, but noted that the real cause of death was inequality.* [5]

The early retired, not yet eligible for Medicare, give us other examples of people without access to affordable care despite their higher income levels. They are healthy people who have always bought their own health insurance, but are now confronted with big premium hikes and high cost sharing without being able to qualify for tax credits under the ACA. [6]

Teri Goodrich, 59, and her husband, John Kistle, 57, of Raleigh, North Carolina bought health insurance through their state's exchange for three years, but cancelled their insurance when premiums reached $19,200 a year with deductibles of $7,500 each. They later purchased short-term coverage, non-compliant with the ACA, for limited catastrophic coverage. As they said, 'We're getting slammed. We didn't budget for this.' [7]

2. The underinsured

Even with the ACA, we already have an epidemic of underinsurance in this country with 31 million people finding themselves without coverage when they need it despite paying more every year for premiums, deductibles, copayments, coinsurance, and out-of-pocket costs. The Commonwealth Fund defines underinsurance as households spending 10 percent or more of their annual income on medical care (not including premiums). It has also found that more than two of five underinsured Americans cannot afford to seek needed health care. [8] Under the Trump administration's stealth sabotage of the ACA, the word "insurance" will become meaningless. Even if "insured" with a short-term or bronze plan, people will be worse off than ever, especially because health care costs will continue to soar unabated in a deregulated marketplace.

3. Can't afford health insurance

As we saw in the last chapter, premiums in 2019 are expected to go up by more than 60 percent in some states, with an average of an 18 percent increase across the country. But these premiums will buy less and less coverage. Insurers will entice some people to buy junk policies by offering them at low premiums, but the protection they will provide will be minimal and not qualify as actual insurance.

Here is what two middle class families in Charlottesville, Virginia, found when they went shopping for coverage on HealthCare. gov in November 2017:

> *Sara Stovall, 40, does customer-support work for a small software company. After researching her options on HealthCare.gov, she found that premiums for her family of four would triple to $3,000 a month with a deductible of $12,000, way beyond her ability to pay. She had been a believer in the ACA, but said 'It's not working as it was supposed to. It's being sabotaged, and I feel like a pawn.'*

> *Ian Dixon, 38, works as a developer of mobile apps. Even though he does not need an assistant, he has considered hiring an employee just so he could buy health insurance as a small business at a cost less than what he and his family would pay on their own. He found two options on HealthCare.gov: (1) a plan with premiums of about $37,000 a year, with a deductible of $9,200 a year; or (2) a plan with annual premiums of $30,000 with a higher deductible of $14,400 a year.* [9]

4. Cost sharing too high

Cost sharing with enrollees in health insurance plans has been a long-held mantra among conservatives, believing that patients with "more skin in the game" will be more conscious of costs and make more prudent decisions about their own health care. This premise has been completely disproven by experience over decades as ineffective in containing health care costs. But the disproven belief continues in TrumpCare with deductibles, copayments and other forms of cost sharing still widespread through the insurance market, even in privatized public programs.

Paul Melquist and his wife in St. Paul, Minnesota are both 59. Paul worked in the defense industry and retired at the end of 2016. He delayed his retirement due to rising costs of health insurance, but was shocked to find they are even worse than he'd imagined. They pay $15,000 a year in premiums for a bronze plan with the first $6,550 for each of them for health care expenses out-of-pocket. So they end up having to pay out some $30,000 a year before anything gets covered. As Paul says, 'It's not that my life is falling apart, but the Affordable Care Act has ruined a lot of things I'd like to have done, [including being better able to help pay for his grandchildren's college expenses].' [10]

The cruel downside of increasing cost sharing is illustrated by the recent, possibly preventable death, of an elementary school teacher in Weatherford, Texas.

Heather Holland, 38-year old married mother of two, fell ill with what was thought to be the flu, but did not pick up a flu medication because she felt the $116 copay was too high. Her symptoms worsened several days later, she ended up in the ICU, was put on dialysis, and died about two days later. [11]

Although we can never know whether the medication could have prevented her death in this instance, we do know that many patients delay or forgo needed care because of high cost sharing and incur worse outcomes.

5. Seniors having trouble affording care

Although Medicare has been a solid rock for more than 50 years in what has become a volatile and unstable health insurance market in this country, seniors still have trouble affording their health care costs. Seniors' out-of-pocket spending consumed 41 percent of Medicare beneficiaries' per capita Social Security income, on average, in 2013. [12] One in four seniors have problems getting care because of costs. [13]

The GOP and Trump administration will make these problems markedly worse, again mostly by administrative policies led by CMS. Seema Verma, head of CMS, has long been a proponent of privatizing Medicare, as has House Speaker Paul Ryan. They would like to convert traditional Medicare into a voucher program, eliminating the long-standing social contract with the elderly for universal access to care. The administration has already changed its premium policy to allow insurers to charge seniors five times as much as younger people, not the 3:1 ratio set by the ACA. Under a voucher system, private insurers could tailor their benefits to attract younger and healthier seniors, leaving sicker seniors in a higher risk pool with much higher costs, thereby threatening a death spiral for traditional Medicare. [14]

6. Restrictive Medicaid changes

With repeal and replacement of the ACA sidelined, at least for now, more states are requesting waivers from DHHS to implement their own policies, which may include work requirements, imposing premiums, lockout from coverage for non-payment or not updating changes in income quickly enough, and lifetime limits for Medicaid eligibility, perhaps for three to five years. These kinds of waivers have already been approved in Kentucky, Indiana, and Arkansas. [15] The work requirement is particularly regressive in that most Medicaid beneficiaries are already working; many who don't are caregivers, in school, unable to work because of illness or disability, or can't find a job in their area.

All of these changes will have more adverse outcomes if Trump's proposed budget cut of almost half a trillion dollars over the next ten years takes effect for the three pillars of the social safety net: Medicaid, federal housing assistance, and SNAP, the food stamp program. According to the Center on Budget and Policy Priorities, there are an estimated 5.7 million Americans that will be put at risk of hunger or homelessness if these budget cuts go forward. Here is what that means for one family struggling to stay afloat.

Daisy Franklin, a 60-year old grandmother in Norwalk, Connecticut, with her household of four, relies on Medicaid, a federal housing voucher, and more than $300 a month in food stamps. She had worked for decades assembling electronic components for local manufacturers, but had to stop after developing fibromyalgia. She now is on disability, collecting $1,250 a month, and cares for her adult daughter's two young children while she supplements the household income with a $10 an hour part-time job. Even with the disability check, food stamps, and a housing voucher that covers two-thirds of their $1,450 a month rent, their money is close to running out at the end of the month. As Daisy says: 'There's a lot of families in our same boat. People are afraid. They don't know what's going to happen to them.' [16]

7. Annual and lifetime limits

The costs of today's high-tech medicine has put many of us at risk for enormous costs that can lead to our bankruptcy for a single major illness or accident. Many insurers are setting annual and lifetime limits for coverage. It may at first seem that a $1 million lifetime limit would be enough, but it will not turn out that way for many patients and families in today's market of runaway costs.

8. Trouble paying medical bills

In 2016, one-third of non-elderly Americans reported problems paying their medical bills, which are now the most common reason for receiving a debt collection phone call. There is now a large and growing debt collection industry that often results in the arrest and jailing of many patients, with little protection from state courts and local prosecutors.

According to a recent report from the ACLU, *A Pound of Flesh: The Criminalization of Private Debt*, one in five Americans has unpaid medical bills that have gone to collection. There are more than 6,000 debt collection agencies operating in the country, collecting billions of dollars each year. The ACLU has found instances in which threatening letters have been sent for bounced checks as low as $2.00. The criminalization of private debt happens when judges issue arrest warrants for people who failed to appear in court, often when they were unaware of receiving such notice. Many people miss their court dates because of work, childcare responsibilities, physical disability, illness, lack of transportation, or because they didn't receive notice of their court date. Although Congress abolished debtors' prisons in 1833, look at what is going on today. [17]

Here are just two examples of how extreme this problem has become:

> *Denise Zencka, mother of three, was arrested in Indiana in 2013 for non-payment of medical bills incurred from cancer treatment. She lived with her parents in Florida for several months during her recovery, during which— unbeknownst to her—she had been ordered to appear in small-claims court in Indiana. Three arrest warrants were issued when she failed to appear. She had already filed for*

bankruptcy when she was arrested and jailed—in a men's mental health unit because she was physically unable to climb the stairs to the women's section. [18]

A Georgia woman was arrested while caring for her terminally ill mother. She had a 6-yeart old rental debt that her landlord claimed she owed after evicting her from her trailer home. She was jailed overnight. Her mother died two days later. [19]

Declining Access due to Inequality

Inequality within our population has been increasing at an ever-faster rate in recent years. Today, in this land of plenty with a federal budget nearly $3.5 trillion, there are 43 million Americans living in poverty out of our population of 326 million. [20] According to a recent report from Heather Boushey, Executive Director of the Washington Center for Equitable Growth, almost two-thirds of tax cuts from the GOP's tax bill of 2017 go to the top 20 percent. The top 1 percent of earners in 1980 took in 27 times more income than the bottom 50 percent. Since then that multiple has tripled to at least 80. [21]

The growing proportion of our society with limited incomes is increasingly vulnerable to worse health outcomes due to declining access to care. As Dr. David Ansell, former chief of general medicine at Cook County Hospital in Chicago for 17 years and author of *The Death Gap: How Inequality Kills*, says of his 40 years in medicine:

Our current multi-payer for-profit health insurance system perpetuates premature death by putting many people at an extreme disadvantage when it comes to affording care. Those who have better health insurance policies can access better care. However, even patients with insurance cards face skyrocketing copays, deduct-ibles and pharmaceutical prices that keep them from seeking care. Last year, 27 percent of Americans said they had postponed or avoided getting care they needed because of the cost; 23 percent said they had skipped a recommended test or treatment due to cost; and 21 percent said they had chosen not to fill prescriptions for medication because they couldn't afford it. . . . Death rates tell the same story. Since 1980, there have been dramatic gains in life expectancy for the top 20 percent of U. S. earners. At the same time, the poorest 20 per-cent have seen their life expectancy plummet. [22]

Concluding comment:

As Dr. Angell observes in her opening quote, this situation is immoral.

Michael Corcoran of *Truthout* adds this important conclusion:

Until the United States adopts a model of social insurance that provides health care to all, regardless of income, the poor will continue to be treated like collateral damage in the war against equality and justice. [23]

This chapter has shown us how TrumpCare will become an unmitigated disaster for much of our population, all under the lie that we will see better care for all of us! As we will see in the next chapter, having "health insurance" has become more and more volatile and inadequate.

References:

1. Angell, M. The benefits of Bernie Sanders' 'Medicare for All' plan. *Boston Globe*, September 21, 2017.

2. U. S. Census Bureau, September 2017.

3. Collins. SR et al. How the Affordable Care Act has improved Americans' ability to buy health insurance on their own. *Commonwealth Fund*, February 1, 2017.

4. Auter, Z. U. S. uninsured rate rises to 12.3 percent in third quarter. *Gallup News*, October 20, 2017.

5. Ansell, D. I watched my patients die of poverty for 40 years. It's time for single payer. *The Washington Post*, September 13, 2017.

6. Rovner, J. Overlooked by ACA: Many people paying full price for insurance 'getting slammed.' *Kaiser Health News*, October 9, 2017.

7. Ibid # 6.

8. Issue Brief. The problem of underinsurance and how rising deductibles will make it worse. Findings from the Commonwealth Fund Biennial Health Insurance Survey, 2014. *The Commonwealth Fund*, May 20, 2015.

9. Pear, R. Middle-class families confront soaring health insurance costs. *New York Times*, November 16, 2017.

10. Ibid # 6.

11. Coyne, C, Gibson, J. Weatherford teacher dies from flu effects. *Weatherford Democrat*, February 5, 2018.

12. Cubanski, J, Neuman, T, Smith, KE. Medicare beneficiaries' out-of-pocket health care spending as a share of income now and projections for the future. *Kaiser Family Foundation*, January 2018.

13. Osborn. R, Doty, MM, Moulds, D et al. Older Americans were sicker and faced more financial barriers to health care than counterparts in other countries. *Health Affairs*, November 15, 2017.

14. Richtman, M. GOP's proposed Medicare voucher program would lead to demise of the system. *The Hill*, March 5, 2018.

15. Bernstein, J, Katch, H. Trump administration's under the radar attack on Medicaid is picking up speed. *The Washington Post*, March 6, 2018.

16. Dewey, C, Jan, T. 'We would literally not survive': How Trump's plans for the social safety net would affect America's poorest. *The Washington Post*, February 14, 2018.

17. Turner, J. *A Pound of Flesh: The Criminalization of Private Debt.* *American Civil Rights Union*, 2018.

18. Germanos, A. New report details how Americans who have debt held by collection agencies can get thrown in jail. *Common Dreams*, February 21, 2018.

19. Rozsa, M. Courts are manipulated by private debt collectors. *The Progressive Populist*, March 15, 2018, p. 9.

20. Powers, N. Fear of a black planet: Under the Republican push for welfare cuts, racism boils. *Truthout*, January 21, 2018.

21. Boushey, H. The tax bill should've been called the Inequality Exacerbation Act of 2017. *The Hill*, December 22, 2017.

22. Ansell, D. I watched my patients die of poverty for 40 years. It's time for single payer. *The Washington Post,* September 13, 2017.

23. Corcoran, M. A legal battle is mounting against the GOP's attack on Medicaid. *Truthout*, February 6, 2018.

CHAPTER 9

INADEQUACY AND INSTABILITY
OF COVERAGE

Right-wing corporate-funded ideologues have fabricated a new negative notion of "freedoms" derived from individual choice. You're free to be poor, free to be politically powerless or free to be ill and uncared for — it's all a matter of decisions you freely make in life, and our larger society has no business interfering with your free will.

—Jim Hightower, author of the *Hightower Lowdown* [1]

The above quote says it all about the devious promises of TrumpCare. In previous times, having health insurance gave one some level of protection against the costs of unpredictable illness and accidents. No more, as we shall see in this chapter. Here we have two goals: (1) to describe various ways in which insurance under TrumpCare is inadequate; and (2) to discuss other ways that make this insurance unstable and unreliable.

Inadequate Health Insurance

Here are four ways that belie Trump's promise of "great insurance for everyone."

1. Copper plans

One of the provisions of the Murray-Alexander bill in the Senate in the fall of 2017 called for allowing all individuals to purchase lower premium copper plans in the individual market. The bill failed at the time, but may resurface in 2018 as a supposed way to deal with soaring health insurance premiums. Although the premiums for copper plans may be attractively low, they cover only 50 percent of health care costs and had an average deductible of $7,150 in 2017. These spartan catastrophic plans are no answer to the needs of patients and families for real health insurance, and run counter to the physical and financial well being of those supposedly "insured." [2]

2. Short-term plans

After just three weeks on the job as head of DHHS, Alex Azar proposed expansion of short-term plans that are exempt from the ACA's consumer protections that were discussed in the last chapter. The ACA limited short-term plans to just three months; Azar's proposal extended them to 12 months while eliminating the ACA's requirement for coverage of all ten essential health benefits. Short-term plans were once intended to be a brief gap-filler for people between jobs or for college students taking a semester off. But the Trump administration is now using them as another way to get around the ACA's patient protections. Azar framed this "advance" as being "all about choice, it's about options for more individuals." [3]

3. Junk insurance

Perhaps the most important threat to patients' insurance coverage is the elimination of the ACA's requirement to cover all ten essential health benefits. This requirement resulted from pre-ACA days when insurers could market policies that fell far short of patients' needs, who often didn't understand what their plans wouldn't cover. Here is one patient's experience from those times:

Ned Scott, 34, in Tucson, Arizona had a health plan before the ACA that left him with $40,000 to $50,000 in unpaid medical bills after he developed testicular cancer in his late 20s. Once he learned that he needed coverage, he discovered that the plan limited outpatient care to just $2,000 a year, and failed to cover all of his treatment from chemotherapy to CT scans. [4]

Under TrumpCare, insurers can again deny coverage for pre-existing conditions. It is estimated that 130 million Americans have one or another pre-existing conditions that could leave them uninsured. Millions more are diagnosed with new illnesses every year that could also render them uninsurable in these times. Andy Slavitt, former Acting Administrator of CMS from 2015 to January 2017, raises these concerns about "junk insurance:"

- *Consumers who purchase these junk policies are going to be putting themselves at risk, both medically and financially. . . . Junk insurance would reverse the precipitous decline in medical bankruptcies that has occurred since the ACA took effect.*
- *For insurance companies, this is a license to steal. Limiting cancer coverage may attract more people with lower premiums, but it will prevent paying out those costly claims.*
- *Insurance will become gradually less available, particularly for expensive conditions.* [5]

4. Unaffordable cost sharing

In order to discourage "frivolous" use of care (and of course to raise revenues for their shareholders!), insurers are often raising their cost sharing requirements. This example gives us a sense of what is going on.

Ali Carlin, 28, used to see her therapist in Richmond,
Virginia every week paying a copayment of $25 per ses-
sion. But her therapist stopped accepting her insurance
in 2015 and increased her copay to $110 per session. In
Virginia, one-quarter of behavioral office visits are out-
of-network, more than seven times more than for medical
care. Although Ali has an annual income of $30,000, she
says that she can't afford the out-of-pocket costs of a ther-
apist or psychiatrist for care of her borderline personality
disorder and addiction issues. As she says: 'I just can't
afford it. I'm choosing groceries over a therapist.' [6]

Insurers have targeted supposed overuse of emergency rooms on the basis that many ER visits are avoidable. A recent national study, however, found that only 3.3 percent of ER visits were "avoidable" in not needing hospital admission, diagnostic or screening services, procedures, or medications. Many "avoidable" visits were for substance abuse, mental health, or dental conditions that usually require care. [7]

Unstable Health Insurance
1. Denial of services

Insurers increasingly deny services by whatever means they can in order to bolster their financial bottom lines. Aetna, the third largest insurer in the country with some 22 million enrollees, has recently drawn scrutiny for one of its medical directors acknowledging that he denied payment for medical care without any review of patients' medical records. This is what happened to one patient:

Gillen Washington was a student at Northern Arizona
University in 2014 when Aetna denied authorization for

the costly drug infusion he'd been receiving every month to treat his rare immunodeficiency disease. He appealed, but while waiting for a decision he was hospitalized with pneumonia and a collapsed lung. During the lawsuit that followed, the medical director admitted that he didn't look at patients' medical records in order to make coverage decisions, instead relying on information provided by nurses, as he claimed he had been trained to do. [8, 9]

In the aftermath of this report, Aetna's prior-authorization practices are being investigated in six states. [10]

2. Changing and narrowing networks

Narrowing networks is another tool used by private insurers to enhance their business model rather than to improve service to patients. Insurers try to attract enrollees by offering lower premiums rather than wider networks. Their decisions about networks have nothing to do with quality. When patients are selecting a health plan, they generally compare plans by premiums and cost sharing requirements, but they have very little opportunity to determine whether physicians, other providers, or hospitals of their choice are in an insurer's network. That information is often inaccurate, outdated, or even wrong. Networks can be changed with little notice, whereby even physicians and patients are unaware of the change.

A narrow network has been defined as having less that 25 percent of physicians, hospitals, and other providers within a network. A few states, such as California and Washington, try to regulate the adequacy of networks, but mostly regulation is lax. It has become even more so as the Trump administration leaves all oversight to the states without any federal guidance.

Here are two examples of this problem, which has a lot to do with patients' costs of care when they need out-of-network care. [11]

> *Cynthia Harvey in Spokane, Washington, bought health insurance from Coordinated Care, after reading a brochure promising a robust roster of physicians and coverage of a wide range of services, including emergency room care. Despite the brochure, there were no in-network emergency room physicians, leaving her with a $1,544 bill from an out-of-network ER physician when she needed care.*

> *Steven Milman, a periodontist in Austin, Texas, chose Superior Health, owned by the same parent company as Coordinated Care, the Centene Corporation, after reading on its website that the Austin Diagnostic Clinic, with 140 physicians, was in its network. After he was enrolled, Steven found out that the Austin Diagnostic Clinic was no longer accepting Superior patients, a decision that had been made months earlier. After a lengthy delay and repeated requests, he was finally assigned to a primary care physician, who was an obstetrician-gynecologist! A class action lawsuit has been filed against Centene over the issue of network provider adequacy.*

A 2016 national study puts numbers on the extent of this problem. It found that the average network for ACA plans included just 24 percent of all primary care providers in a given area, more than twice the proportion of mental health care providers. [12]

3. Insurers exiting markets

Insurers leave markets when they become insufficiently profitable, often without much advance notice. The serious impacts of these exits on patients and families are well illustrated by these two examples: [13]

> *Four-year-old Colette Briggs from Loudoun County in Virginia has been receiving intermittent spinal tap chemotherapy and emergency care for an aggressive leukemia over the last two years at Inova Fairfax Hospital. The family has purchased health insurance from Anthem for years, but in 2017 decided to stop selling plans in Virginia. Under pressure from the state, it returned to some counties and cities in Virginia, but not to Loudoun County. The only option for the family was Cigna, but it does not cover Fairfax Hospital, the only local hospital with a dedicated pediatric cancer unit. Christopher, Colette's father, a self-employed communications consultant for nonprofit groups, spent the next two months trying to figure out how to get alternate coverage, without success so far. He considered moving the family to another county in Virginia that offers Anthem coverage or to another state which has a top-tier pediatric hospital.*
>
> *Anthem also did not re-enter the market in Henrico County, just outside of Richmond, where Cindy Jones lives and works as Virginia's director for Medicaid. Even with her connections, she has faced the same predicament as the Briggs family. Her adult son, Daniel Bowling, was diagnosed two years earlier with leukemia. He had been living and working in Myrtle Beach, South Carolina, but at age 27 moved home so that his mother could care for him and where he could receive treatments at Virginia Commonwealth University. That is—until he*

found that his insurance (Anthem) would not cover care there. Desperate to find coverage for Daniel, Cindy even considered quitting her job and moving with her son to North Carolina, where he could receive care at Duke University Hospital.

4. Lost coverage due to dis-enrollment

Private Medicare Advantage plans economize by providing less needed as well as more unneeded care. On the lesser side, compared to traditional Medicare, they provide 24.4 percent fewer diagnostic tests, 38 percent fewer flu shots, 14.9 percent fewer colon cancer screenings, and 16 percent fewer non-emergent and emergent visits to emergency rooms. [14]

Medicare Advantage plans further increase their revenues by pushing high-cost patients to dis-enroll by charging high copayments for drugs and services, including hospitalization, ambulance services and home health care. [15]

5. Loss of Medicaid coverage by changing eligibility

Many people, especially children, are losing eligibility for Medicaid as states develop more rigorous income and payment requirements under the Trump policy of granting more flexibility to states. Texas has one of the country's strictest Medicaid verification systems, running regular checks of family finances after children are enrolled to ensure that they still qualify. Here is what this means for one family.

Dawn Poole and her husband live near Houston, Texas, where both work in seasonal industries—she as an hourly worker in agriculture and he in oil. Their work hours and incomes often change on a monthly, even weekly basis. They have nine children, all with complex medical problems. They can lose Medicaid coverage one month, then re-qualify the next month. Their children lose necessary health care during these gaps in coverage, even though they remain eligible on an annual basis with their household income less than 138 percent of federal poverty level. [16]

While this rigorous income testing is intended to save the state money and shrink the Medicaid program, this is not a rational policy whether in Texas or across the country. Nationally, children account for more than two-fifths of Medicaid's enrollment but represent less than one-fifth of Medicaid spending. Seniors and people with disabilities account for about one-half of Medicaid spending. The frequent income testing adds a complex and costly administrative burden to states following this practice. [17]

Another way that states can limit eligibility for Medicaid under Trump's new flexibility to states is to impose premiums, then drop coverage for non-payment. Premiums were not part of Medicaid until it was expanded in some states in 2014. Six states have now added premiums in their Medicaid programs, including Indiana, Michigan, Iowa, Montana, Arkansas, and Kentucky. In Arkansas, only 20 percent of the state's Medicaid enrollees paid their $13 monthly premiums in 2017, while tens of thousands of Medicaid enrollees in other states either could not or would not pay their premiums. For many families on Medicaid, even very low premiums meant they had to choose between buying food, paying their electric bill and rent, or pay premiums. [18] So far, Indiana is the only one of these states that will lock enrollees out from coverage for non-payment of premiums.[19]

6.   *Interruptions in private coverage*

Interruptions in private health insurance are not only common but hazardous among adults in the U.S. A recent study of working-age adults with type 1 diabetes found a five-fold increase in the need for acute health care services, lower perceived health status, and lower satisfaction with life. [20]

Concluding comment

These last two chapters have shown how inadequate, expensive and volatile health insurance has become in the U. S. even as the costs of care continue upward at a pace far exceeding the cost of living. In the next chapter, we will examine how containment of these costs is nowhere on the horizon, and is even being exacerbated under TrumpCare.

References:

1.   Hightower, J. The GOP will free you from having health care. *Common Dreams*, June 14, 2017.

2.   McCanne, D. Copper plans are an unacceptable trade-off. Quote of the Day, October 19, 2017.

3.   Azar, A. As quoted by Cunningham, PW. Azar makes his first Obamacare move. *The Washington Post*, February 21, 2018.

4.   Abelson, R. In clash over health bill, a growing fear of 'junk insurance.' *New York Times*, July 15, 2017.

5.   Slavitt, A. Junk insurance plan proves Trump doesn't care about your health. *USA TODAY*, March 5, 2018.

6.   Gold, J. If your insurer covers few therapists, is that really mental health parity? *Kaiser Health News*, November 30, 2017.

7. Hsia, RY, Niedzwieckl, M. Avoidable emergency department visits: A starting point. *International Journal for Quality in Health Care*, August 31, 2017.

8. Editorial Board. What the Aetna scandal tells us about our healthcare system: It's a money pit. *Los Angeles Times*, February 14, 2018.

9. Livingston, S. Two states question Aetna's prior-authorization practices amid CVS merger. *Modern Healthcare*, February 13, 2018.

10. Livingston, S. Six state regulators now scrutinizing Aetna prior-authorization practices. *Modern Healthcare*, February 15, 2018.

11. Ollove, M. Trump administration: Let states decide if health plans have enough doctors. *Pew Charitable Trusts*, February 6, 2018.

12. Zhu, JM, Zhang, Y, Polsky, D. Networks in ACA marketplaces are narrower for mental health than for primary care. *Health Affairs* 36 (9), September, 2017.

13. Itkowitz, C. Parents of a 4-year-old with cancer can't buy ACA plan to cover her hospital care. *The Washington Post*, November 15, 2017.

14. Curto, V, Einav, V, Finklestein, A et al. Healthcare spending and utilization in public and private Medicare. NBER Working Paper 23090, January 2017.

15. Park, S, Basu, A, Coe, N et al. Service-level selection in Medicare Advantage in response to risk adjustment. NBER Working Paper 24038, November 2017.

16. Luthra, S. Seesawing family income threatens kids' Medicaid coverage in Texas. *Kaiser Health News*, June 16, 2017.

17. Ibid # 16.

18. Galewitz, P. Tens of thousands of Medicaid recipients skip paying new premiums. *Kaiser Health News*, March 1, 2018.

19. Galewitz, P. Indiana gets federal approval for Medicaid plan that could slice enrollment. *Kaiser Health News*, February 2, 2018.

20. Rogers, M.A.M. Lee, J.M., Tiperneni, R et al. Interruption in private health insurance and outcomes in adults with Type 1 diabetes: A longitudinal study. *Health Affairs*, July 2018.

CHAPTER 10

LACK OF COST CONTAINMENT

Healthcare will be a lot less expensive for everyone—the
government, consumers, providers.

—President Donald Trump [1]

The above statement, like so many Trump promises, is a bald
lie that shows no awareness of the complexity of health care or the
long history of uncontrolled health care costs in this country. This
is just the latest of lies, which are a bipartisan problem. Before the
ACA was enacted, President Obama promised everyone would save
$2,500 with it and be able to keep their own doctor and insurance, all
of which soon became fiction.

This chapter has three goals: (1) to briefly summarize the history
of rising health care costs over the last 50-plus years; (2) to discuss
the impacts of uncontrolled health care inflation; and (3) to briefly
consider the lessons we should learn from our failure to rein in these
increasingly unaffordable costs.

Relentless Rise of Health Care Costs in the U. S.

When we look back at health care costs in the U. S. since the
1960s, we find a steep, unending increase that defies imagination,
as shown so clearly by Figure 10.1. Over that time period, annual
inflation of the cost of living averaged 3.79 percent [2], but health care
costs far exceeded that. By 2016, per capita health care spending
reached $10,348. [3]

FIGURE 10.1

TOTAL U.S. HEALTH SPENDING
AND MEDICAID SPENDING, 1966-2015

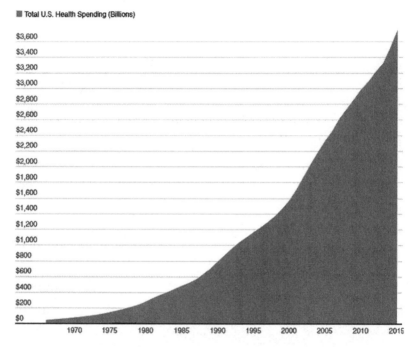

Source: Centers for Medicare & Medicaid Services

Passage of the ACA in 2010 made no dent in this problem, instead exacerbating it. According to CMS, the net cost of health insurance more than doubled by 2013, as did the net cost of administration. [4] Today, the U. S. spends almost twice as much as 10 high-income countries on medical care. In fact, the gap between these countries has grown markedly over the period 1970 and 2016, as documented by Figure 10.2.

Prices of labor and goods, including pharmaceuticals and devices and administrative costs are driving this run-away train.[5] Taking Big PhRMA as an example, about 90 percent of newly approved drugs bring few or no clinical benefits since the FDA does not require added efficacy or safety. Most drug research is aimed to generate new patents of minor variations in order to charge patent protected prices. [6]

Here are just two examples, of many thousands that happen every day, that illustrate the incredible medical bills that patients are being charged, no matter how hard they try to seek out lesser prices.

Elodie Fowler, age 3, had an MRI at Lucile Packard Children's Hospital in Palo Alto, California in 2016 in an attempt to better understand her rare genetic condition that was causing swelling along the right side of her body and problems processing regular food. Having a generous plan from the ACA's exchange, her parents decided to go out-of-network to a clinic that specialized in their daughter's rare condition. That plan would cover one half of a "fair price" MRI. The price tag ended up at $25,000, including $16,632 for the MRI, $4,016 for the anesthesia, $2,703 for a recovery room, plus doctor fees. The insurance covered only $1,547, leaving the family responsible for $23,795. The parents negotiated the bill down to $16,000, and is paying it down in monthly $700 installments. By comparison, the average cost for an MRI in the U. S. is $1,119 vs. $503 in Switzerland and $215 in Australia. [7]

Elizabeth Moreno, 30, had back surgery in late 2015. After surgery, her surgeon prescribed an opioid for pain and what seemed like a follow-up urine drug test. She and her physician father were shocked soon thereafter when they received a bill for $17,850 from a laboratory for the urine test, which checked on all kinds of drugs, including an illegal hallucinogenic drug known as PCP. Her insurer,

Blue Cross and Blue Shield of Texas, refused to cover,
apparently because the lab was out of network, and sent
Elizabeth an explanation of benefits that valued the work
at $100.92. A complaint was filed with the Texas attorney
general's office, but the bill remained. Experts doubted
the need for the test, which was considered fraudulent.
A reporter for Kaiser Health News noted that the testing
boom consumes billions of dollars every year, often for
needless tests at exorbitant prices. [8]

FIGURE 10.2

SINCE 1980, THE GAP HAS WIDENED BETWEEN U.S.
HEALTH SPENDING AND THAT OF OTHER COUNTRIES

Total health expenditures as percent of GDP, 1970-2016

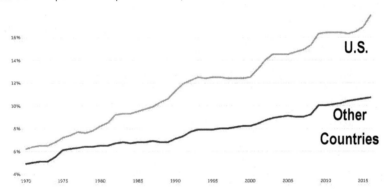

Excludes spending on structures, equipment, and non-commercial medical research. Data unavailable for the Netherlnds for 1970 and 1971; Australia in 1970; Germany in 1991; and France from 1971 through 1974, 1976 through 1979, 1981 through 1985, and 1986 through 1989. These countries are not included in calculated averages for those years. Break in series in 2003 for Belgium and France, and in 2005 for the Netherlands. Data for 2016 are estimated values. The 2016 U.S. value was obtained from National Health Expenditure data.

Source: Kaiser Family Foundation analysis of data from OECD (2017). "OECD Health Data: Health expenditure and financing. Health, health expenditure Indicators", OECD Health Statistics (database) (Accessed on March 19, 2017), • Get the Data • PNG

There have been many theories about why health care costs continue to rise at astronomical levels in this country, including that patients overuse the system at the drop of a hat. That reason is readily discredited by the growing unaffordability of care, the financial barriers to care, and comparative data across other advanced industrial countries that control costs much better than we do while patients access care much more often than we do. According to the Commonwealth Fund, Germans see the doctor 9.9 times a year, Dutch 8 times, and Americans just 4 times a year. [9]

While prices and the lack of significant price controls are the leading reasons for our lack of cost containment, other factors also play a big role. The growth of the medical-industrial complex, incentives throughout our market-based system to maximize profits, consolidation of hospital systems and insurers, increasing bureaucracy and waste in the private sector, and fraud are also parts of the problem. As giant corporate systems buy up hospitals and physicians' practices at an increasing rate, they increase their market share to near-monopoly levels with leeway to set prices to what the traffic will bear. [10] It is estimated that we waste at least $150 billion a year on hospital bureaucracy and another $300 billion on private insurers and the paperwork they impose on physicians. [11] As Gerald Friedman, professor of economics at the University of Massachusetts, Amherst, observes:

> *Administrative complexity and waste are no accident but rather are baked into our private health insurance system and made worse by continuing attempts to use competitive market processes to achieve social ends other than maximizing profit.* [12]

Impacts of Uncontrolled Inflation of Health Care Costs

Confronted with these enormous costs of health care, rising much faster than the costs of living, how can Americans possibly cope with them and receive necessary health care? The answer is, unfortunately, for much of the population, they can't. Even if insured by an average employer-sponsored preferred provider organization (PPO) plan, the cost of health care for a typical American family of four in 2018, according to the Milliman Medical Index, has reached an average of more than $28,000 per year.[13] That consumes almost one-half of the 2017 median household income in the U. S. of $59,358! For comparison, the Commonwealth Fund considers those spending more than 10 percent of their annual income as financial hardship. Figure 10.3 shows the monthly costs of health care for a two-parent, two-child family across the U. S. at a county level in 2017 dollars, according to the Economic Policy Institute.

FIGURE 10.3

FAMILY ACROSS U.S. AT COUNTY LEVEL

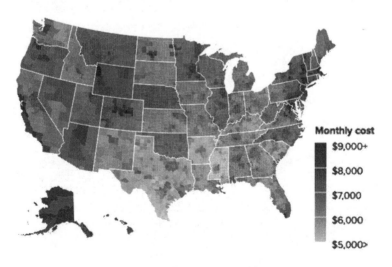

Source: Economic Policy Institute *Family Budget Calculator*, March 2018, Data are in 2017 dollars.

Traditional Medicare has been a rock in rough seas for most seniors since it was enacted in 1965. But even that rock is crumbling, as these markers show.

- Health expenses accounted for an average of 14 percent of household spending among Medicare beneficiaries in 2016 with almost 3 in 10 Medicare households spending more than 20 percent of their household income on health care.[14]
- 37 percent of the average Social Security check now goes toward out-of-pocket health care expenses. [15]
- Cross-national surveys by the Commonwealth Foundation have found that seniors in the U. S. are sicker and face more financial barriers than their counterparts in 10 other high-income countries. [16]
- Long-term care costs are way beyond the reach of most families today, with private nursing home rooms now averaging more than $92,000 per year, Medicare not covering long-term stays, and people having to spend down to Medicaid levels to gain that coverage. [17]
- One-third of the nation's nursing homes have been not-for-profit, but their numbers are declining due to a rising number of their increasingly difficult economic pressures.[18]

And all that even before the intent of the GOP in Congress to cut Medicare and Medicaid.

Takeaway Lessons from Failure to Control Health Care Costs

The U. S. has been an outlier in the world in being totally ineffective in containing health care costs for more than five decades. The ACA has had no real cost containment provisions, while the GOP and Trump administration's policies will be even more lax in this respect. We have an ongoing free-for-all in an unfettered marketplace that places profits to the few over service to the many patients and their families.

What takeaway lessons can we learn from this long-term failure to contain costs? These six stand out:

1.   Free markets do not control costs through competition in health care, as they might in other kinds of markets.

We have been told for decades that competition will work in health care, but long experience tells otherwise. Instead we see increasing consolidation among corporate giants with wide latitude to set prices as they gain market share. Prices are not transparent to the public, be they for hospital services, prescription drugs, or other services. Theoretically, consumers might be able to save money with more information and being savvier shoppers, but this has been proven untrue. A recent study found that less than 7 percent of total health care spending in 2011 was paid by consumers for "shoppable services." [19]

Don Berwick, M.D., former administrator of CMS and founder of the Institute for Healthcare Improvement, has this to say about the situation:

> *I find little evidence anywhere that market forces, bluntly used, that is, consumer choice among an array of products with competitors fighting it out, leads to a health care system you want and need. In the U. S. competition has become toxic: it is a major reason for our duplicative, supply-driven, fragmented health care system . . . Unfettered growth and pursuit of institutional self-interest has been the engine of low-value for the U. S. health care system. It has made it unaffordable, and hasn't helped patients at all.* [20]

2.   *The pervasive business "ethic" to maximize revenues to providers of health care works against the public interest, as does involvement by Wall Street profiteers.*

Recent decades have seen the takeover of the medical-industrial complex by ever-larger corporations with close ties to Wall Street. Physicians and many other health care providers are now employed by large hospital systems or other corporate entities where they are under the thumb of administrators pushing for higher reimbursement. Along the way, the traditional ethic of service has become lost as "shareholder capitalism" holds sway.

Here is one example of corporate greed whereby pharmaceutical companies acquire rare drugs and then make huge price increases.

> *Martin Shkreli started a hedge fund, MSMB, on Wall Street in his 20s. He lobbied the FDA not to approve drugs that he was shorting. He then started a pharmaceutical company, Retrophin, from which he was later fired by its board for allegedly using it as a personal piggy bank to pay back angry investors. At 32 he became CEO of the startup Turing Pharmaceuticals that bought up Daraprim, a 62-year-old drug for treating toxoplasmosis, a life-threatening parasitic infection. It cost less than one dollar to make, and was selling at $13.50 a tablet until Shkreli increased the price by 5,000 percent to $750 a tablet.* [21]

Unfortunately, this is not an isolated example. Of the 25 drugs with the fastest-rising prices between 2013 and 2015, twenty were owned by firms that were involved in hedge fund, private equity or similar speculative attacks during that time. [22]

3. *All of our payment policies have failed to contain costs or improve quality of care.*

Payment experiments adopted by Medicare in recent years were intended to save costs and improve quality of care. But they have clearly failed, even as they increased costs and bureaucracy. As examples, accountable care organizations (ACOs) and the so-called Pay-for-Performance (P4P) programs have produced no savings and little or no improvement in patient outcomes. Most physicians and health policy experts believe the "quality" measures are flawed. Instead, these two programs have increased administrative costs and forced smaller hospitals and physician practices into large corporate systems. [23] Meanwhile, we continue on with a system that provides up to one-third of all health care services that are either inappropriate, unnecessary, or even harmful. [24]

Faced with all of the failures of our system to contain costs despite all attempts and with the projections for ongoing increases that will consume almost 20 percent of GDP by 2026, Seema Verma, current CMS administrator, draws this lame and misguided conclusion:

> *This is yet another call to action for CMS to increase market competition and consumer choice within our programs to help control costs and ensure that our programs are available for future generations.* [25]

4. *We pay much more and get much less than other advanced countries.*

Americans are paying much more for health care, by roughly one-half, but getting less for it. As previously mentioned, they are seeing the doctor much less often, being hospitalized less often, and using fewer health care services. The difference, again, is because of our very high health care costs and financial barriers in seeking care. Neil Brennan, president of the Health Care Cost Institute (HCCI) recently observed:

> *It is time to have a national conversation on the role of price increases in the growth of health care spending. Despite the progress made in recent years on value-based care, the reality is that working Americans are using less care but paying more for it every year. Rising prices, especially for prescription drugs, surgery, and emergency department visits, have been primary drivers of faster growth in recent years.* [26]

5. We need a larger role of government to contain health care costs and ensure universal access to necessary care for all Americans.

In health care, the neoliberal agenda of past and current administrations has failed to contain costs and make health care affordable. Our mostly for-profit, unaccountable market-based system is spinning out of control. Budget cutting, less government, further deregulation, shifting health care to the states, and trickle down economics have not, and will not work. Recent decades have proven that corporate stakeholders in the medical-industrial complex will *never* bring us a health care system that meets the needs of all Americans. We are rapidly approaching a breaking point that now needs fundamental reform, especially in how we finance health care.

We should take heed of this important insight by Joseph Stiglitz, Ph.D., Nobel Laureate in Economics and former chief economist at the World Bank:

> *Markets do not lead to efficient outcomes, let alone outcomes that comport with social justice. As a result, there is often good*

reason for government intervention to improve the efficiency of the market. Just as the Great Depression should have made it evident that the market does not work as well as its advocates claim, our recent Roaring Nineties should have made it self-evident that the pursuit of self-interest does not necessarily lead to overall economic efficiency. [27]

It is long past the time when we should re-build our health care system for the common good, not private gain at the expense of patients and their families. We will discuss how to do that in Chapter 15.

6. *We cannot contain health care costs until we reform our financing system.*

Containment of U. S. health care costs will require a transformational change in how we finance and pay for health care services, together with transition over 15 years from a for-profit system to a not-for-profit service-oriented system. This can and should happen with enactment of expanded and improved Medicare for All legislation in Congress (H. R. 676 in the House and S.1804 in the Senate) that will provide universal access to all necessary health care for all Americans. Such a system of single-payer national health insurance will pay hospitals and other facilities through global operating budgets. Physicians and other health professionals will be paid on a negotiated fee basis. Much of today's bureaucracy and waste will be eliminated with a five-fold reduction in administrative costs. The program can be funded through a progressive system of taxation whereby 95 percent of Americans will pay less than they do now for insurance and care. Projected annual savings of some $616 billion can thereby be achieved, including about $503 billion in administrative overhead and $113 billion in prescription drugs through bulk purchasing. [28]

After study of the experience of France, Germany, the UK, Canada and Japan, T. R. Reid drew this conclusion in his excellent book, *The Healing of America: A Global Quest for Better, Cheaper, and Fairer Health Care*:

> The American system does well when it comes to providing medical care, but has a rotten system for financing that care . . . All the other rich countries have found financing models that cover everybody and they still spend much less than we do. We've ignored those foreign models, partly because of "American exceptionalism"—the notion that the United States has nothing to learn from the rest of the world. [29]

This is what we can learn from Canada, our good neighbor to the north, about its successful containment of health care costs since the early 1970s, when it launched universal health care for its entire population with its single-payer program. Figure 10.4 says it all.

FIGURE 10.4

HEALTH COSTS AS % OF GDP
U.S. & Canada, 1960-2014

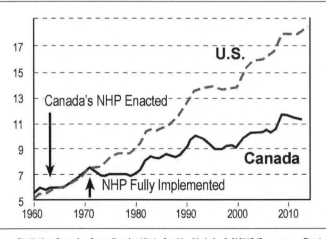

Source: Statistics Canada, Canadian Institute for Health Info & NCHS/Commerce Dept.

Concluding comment

Bad as our health care costs are, they will get worse under Trump's policies of deregulation, industry friendly policies, and deceptive rhetoric. His opening quote to this chapter has no credibility at all—just another blatant lie.

What we now have in health care is a disaster—socially unjust and completely unsustainable. In the next chapter, we'll see how much variability to expect from one state to another, made worse by the policy of the GOP and Trump administration to shift responsibility for health care from the federal government to the states.

References:

1. Trump, DJ. As quoted by Jackson, H C. 6 promises Trump made about health care. *Politico*, March 13, 2017.

2. Calculation using Dr. Petrosino's Education Project, February 17, 2016.

3. Alonzo-Zaldivar, R. Health: $10,345 per person: U. S. health care reaches a new peak. *Association Press*, July 16, 2016.

4. Centers for Medicare and Medicaid Services, Office of the Actuary, National Health Statistics Group. *Health Affairs*, October 2013.

5. Papanicolas, I, Woskie, LR, Jha, AK. Health care spending in the United States and other high-income countries. *JAMA*, March 13, 2018.

6. Light, DW, Caplan, AL. Trump blames free riding foreign states for high U. S. drug prices. *British Medical Journal*, March 16, 2018.

7. Kliff, S. The problem is the prices. *VOX*, October 16, 2017.

8. Schulte, F. Pain hits after surgery when a doctor's daughter is stunned by $17,850 urine test. *Kaiser Health News*, February 16, 2018.

9. Ibid # 7.

10. Fulton, BD. Health and market competition trends in the United States: Evidence and policy responses. *Health Affairs*, September 2017.

11. PNHP press release. Bureaucracy consumes one-quarter of U. S. hospitals' budgets, twice as much as in other nations. *Physicians for a National Health Program*. Chicago. September 8, 2014.

12. Friedman, G. Why market competition has not brought down health care costs. *Truthout*, July 4, 2017.

13. Girod, C, Hart, S, Waltz, S. *2018 Milliman Medical Index*.

14. Cubanski, J, Orgera, K, Neuman, T. The financial burden of health care spending: Larger for Medicare households than for non-Medicare households. Issue Brief. *Kaiser Family Foundation*, March 1, 2018.

15. Phelan, M. How drug prices destroy Social Security benefits, *Social Security Works*. March 29, 2017.

16. Osborn, R, Doty, M, Moulds, D et al. Older Americans were sicker and faced more financial barriers to health care than counterparts in other countries. New York. *Commonwealth Fund*, November 15, 2017.

17. Associated Press. Study: Costs for most long-term care keep climbing. *New York Times*, May 10, 2016, 2017.

18. Flynn, M. Skilled nursing pressures forcing non-profits to sell or close. *Skilled Nursing News*, January 28, 2018.

19. Andrews, M. Consumer choices have limited impact on U. S. health care spending: Study. *Kaiser Health News*, March 4, 2016.

20. Berwick, D. A transatlantic review of the NHS at 60. *British Medical Journal* 337 (7663): 212-214, 2008.

21. Pollack, A. Drug goes from $13.50 a tablet to $750 overnight. *New York Times*, September 20, 2015.

22. Hedge funds attack American health care. *Hedge Clippers*, September 30, 2015.

23. Woolhandler, S, Himmelstein, DU. New prospects for single-payer activists: Swimming in the mainstream . . . with sharks. *Physicians for a National Health Program*. Chicago, IL, Winter 2018 Newsletter, pp. 14-16.

24. Wenner, JB, Fisher, ES, Skinner, JS. Geography and the debate over Medicare reform. *Health Affairs Web Exclusive* W-103, February 13, 2002.

25. Verma, S. CMS Office of the Actuary releases 2017-2026 projections for national health expenditures. Centers for Medicare & Medicaid Services, February 14, 2018.

26. Hellman, J. Study: Americans using less health care, but paying more for it. *The Hill*, January 23, 2018.

27. Stiglitz, JE. Evaluating economic change. *Daedalus* 133/3, Summer, 2004.

28. Friedman, G. Funding H. R. 676: The Expanded and Improved Medicare for All Act. How We Can Afford a National Single-Payer Health Plan. *Physicians for a National Health Program*. Chicago, IL, July 31, 2013.

29. Reid, TR. *The Healing of America: A Global Quest for Better, Cheaper, and Fairer Health Care*. New York. *The Penguin Press*, 2009: pp. 225-226.

CHAPTER 11

PROFITEERING AND LOWER
QUALITY OF CARE

Profiteering in our market-based system has long been a problem, well before and since the ACA was enacted eight years ago. As we have seen in earlier chapters, it is enabled by consolidation of corporate stakeholders, increasing privatization, deregulation and lack of price controls. The efforts by the Trump administration to further deregulate the system and shift health policy to the states will only increase the problem, together with the always-associated impact on lowering the quality of health care.

This chapter has two goals: (1) to give an overview of how TrumpCare continues to encourage profiteering by private insurers, Medicare and Medicaid, the drug industry and other health care providers, with resulting lower quality of care; and (2) to describe how previous efforts to rearrange incentives within the system have failed to improve quality.

Profiteering in health care

Corporatization and growth of for-profit health care in the United States have been rapidly increasing since the 1970s, and Wall Street soon became enamored with profits to be made. Their corporate profits after taxes increased by more than 100 times between 1965 and 1990, at a rate almost 20 times greater than profits of all U. S. corporations. [1]

After his long and expensive encounter with our health care system as a patient and investigative reporter, William Rivers Pitt, senior editor and lead columnist at *Truthout* and author of *The Greatest Sedition Is Silence*, brings us this insight. [2]

> *The problem is that health care in the United States is a for-profit industry, like petroleum speculation or automobile manufacture. It's a few people making a lot of money off of sick people, and after so many years of this being the status quo, they have the political system wired to keep it that way.*

Passage of the ACA did nothing to rein in this long trend to maximize corporate profits rather than service to patients, as Figure 11.1 clearly shows. In fact, CEOs of the largest U. S. health care companies have taken in almost $10 billion since 2010. Leading this list, John Martin, the former CEO of Gilead Sciences, which makes HIV and hepatitis C drugs, accounted for $900 million. [3] This was predicted by Tom Scully, former administrator of CMS in the George W. Bush administration, in these words:

> *Obamacare is not a government takeover of medicine. It is the privatization of health care . . . It is going to make some people very rich.* [4]

A short tour through parts of our system gives us a sense of how private insurers, private Medicare Advantage, privatized Medicaid, the drug industry, some entrepreneurial physicians, and other health care providers manipulate the system to their own self-interest.

FIGURE 11.1

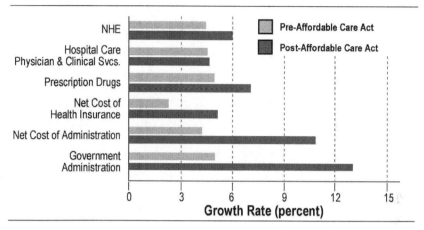

2014 Growth Rates by Selected Sector, Before and After the Impact of the Affordable Care Act

Source: Centers for Medicaid Services, Office of the Actuary, National Health Statistics Group

Insurers

- The second-quarter 2017 profit of Aetna, the country's third largest private insurer, jumped by 52 percent even as it scaled back ACA coverage. [5]

- The consulting firm Avalere Health estimates that 2019 premiums will go up by 69 percent in Iowa, 65 percent in Wyoming, and 64 percent in Utah. [6]

- Insurers have been gaming the ACA's risk-coding program, under which they are paid more by covering older and sicker enrollees, by overstating their health risks. [7]

- In the aftermath of the two-year omnibus spending bill that dropped cost-sharing reduction payments (CSR) and a $30 billion reinsurance program, health insurers are planning major premium increases as they consider whether or not to participate in the 2019 individual market. [8]

- Profit margins of several top insurers for the first quarter of 2018 were the highest in a decade; all six of the largest insurers paid their CEOs more than $17 million in 2017. [9]
- According to a national study by Covered California, cumulative premium increases from 2019 to 2021 will range from 35 percent to more than 90 percent. [10]

Private Medicare Advantage

- Sicker patients on Medicare Advantage plans frequently have to leave their plans for traditional Medicare as insurers cut access to preferred physicians, hospitals, and necessary drug treatment. [11]
- Federal audits of 37 Medicare Advantage plans have found overspending due to inflated risk scores that overstate the severity of such conditions as diabetes and depression for a majority of patients treated. [12]
- A 2015 report by the Commonwealth Fund found that 97 percent of markets for private Medicare Advantage plans in U. S. counties were "highly concentrated" with little competition. [13]

Privatized Medicaid

- Centene Corp., the largest Medicaid insurer in the country, took in $1.1 billion in profits between 2014 and 2016 in California, even as its plans were among the worst performing in the state. [14]
- Overpayments to private Medicaid managed care plans are widespread in more than 30 states, often involving unnecessary, duplicative payments to providers and calling for more scrutiny by auditors. [15]
- Tennessee Medicaid plans, operated by Blue Cross Blue Shield of Tennessee, UnitedHealthcare, and Anthem, are

typical of the poor service of private Medicaid plans, with inadequate physician networks, long waits for care, and denials of many treatments, even as the insurers take in new profits. [16]

Doctor-owned hospitals and facilities

- Physician-owned specialty hospitals that focus on well-reimbursed services, such as in cardiovascular disease and orthopedic surgery, have become common over the last 30 years as a means for physicians to evade laws prohibiting them from referring patients to hospitals in which they are invested. They typically cherry pick well insured patients and maximize revenue as they claim greater efficiency and value. [17]

- Physician-ownership of CT and other imaging centers order two to eight times as many imaging procedures as those not owned by physicians, leading to an estimated $40 billion worth of unnecessary imaging each year. [18]

Free-standing ERs

- The numbers of stand-alone ERs, unattached to hospitals, have been growing in recent years, especially in more affluent areas. Their charges are often four to five times higher than urgent care centers, and patients needing hospitalization or surgery still have to be transported by ambulance to access such care. [19]

Drug industry

- Big PhRMA uses a number of approaches to maximize its profits, including often misleading direct to consumer advertising (banned in many countries), lobbying against any price controls and importation of drugs from other countries, and non-rigorous "research" conducted for marketing purposes. The five largest pharmaceutical companies took in more than $50 billion in profits in 2015.[20]

- Several wholesale drug distributors contributed to the spiraling opioid crisis by shipping huge volumes of prescription opioids to targeted corrupt physicians and pharmacists engaged in a lucrative black market. As one example, a mid-size Ohio-based distributor, Miami-Linken, sent 11 million doses of oxycodone and hydrocodone to Mingo, a rural county in West Virginia with a population of just 25,000. [21] A powerful backlash from industry was then successful in getting legislators in Congress to pass unanimously a bill that made it almost impossible for a weakened DEA to freeze suspicious shipments of opioids.[22]

Nursing homes

- About two-thirds of the nation's 16,000 nursing homes are for profit, with more than one-half owned and controlled by corporate chains. They typically cut nursing staffing to increase revenues resulting in worse patient outcomes. [23]

Home care

- Three-fourths of the country's home health agencies are for-profit, which have been demonstrated to have higher costs and lower quality of care than their not-for-profit counterparts. [24]

Behavioral health

- For-profit behavioral health care, especially substance abuse treatment, is growing and consolidating rapidly, attracting more investors but underserving vulnerable populations. [25, 26]

Hospice

- End of life care through hospice has become a $17 billion industry, with most hospices for profit; they generally spend less on nursing per patient than their not-for-profit counterparts, resulting in worse quality of care and many patients dropping out. [27]

Previous attempts to improve quality of care have failed.

There have been various efforts in recent years to rein in overutilization of health care services as incentivized by our revenue-driven market-based system. The concept of achieving more value and less volume of services has been a goal of such approaches as pay-for-performance (P4P) report cards for physicians and Medicare's accountable care organizations (ACOs). More than 150 quality measures are now in use for outpatient services, such as rates for screening mammography. But most physicians find these "quality" measures neither accurate nor useful and overly burdensome on their practices, while also not effective in improving quality of care. [28]

Both approaches have been dismal failures in controlling costs and improving quality of care. Physicians (and their employers if employed by hospital systems) can easily game the system by cherry picking patients and populations to be cared for. Since socioeconomic factors play a large role in worse outcomes of care, physicians and ACOs are penalized for caring for poorer and disadvantaged patients and populations, while those that avoid their care receive bonus "quality" reimbursement. Although ACOs have grown from 27 participants in 2012 to 561 today, they have failed to produce savings and have even increased federal spending by $384 million from 2013 to 2016. [29] Dr. Karen Joynt Maddox, a cardiologist and health services researcher at Washington University School of Medicine in St. Louis, notes that physicians who serve poor and sicker patients lose out in this program. As she says:

> *We are literally taking money from providers that serve the poor and giving it to providers that serve the rich.* [30]

Markers of failure to improve quality of care

Here are some markers of where we stand now in terms of unacceptable quality of care in this country.

- Up to one-half of medical procedures that are provided by physicians each year are not supported by best scientific evidence. [31]
- Medical errors account for about 250,000 deaths a year. [32]
- A two-year study by the ECRI Institute, a non-profit research group that studies patient safety, found that more than 7,600 so-called wrong-patient errors occurred at 181 health care organizations between 2013 and 2015. [33]
- A 2012 report by the Centers for Disease Control and Prevention (CDC) estimated that 45,000 Americans were dying each year for lack of health insurance; [34] this number would increase significantly under GOP plans that would increase the numbers of uninsured and underinsured.
- The American Academy of Pediatrics calls poverty the most serious chronic disease that children have, often leading to stunted cognitive development, impaired immune function, and psychiatric disorders. [35]
- According to a 2017 study of all states conducted by the Commonwealth Fund, these conclusions were drawn:

1. Across all measures (health care access, quality, avoidable hospital use and costs, health outcomes, and health care equity), there was a three-fold variation in performance, on average, between top- and bottom-performing states.

2. States that expanded Medicaid under the ACA saw greater gains in access to care.

3. Premature death rates crept up in almost two-thirds of states.

4. Disparities within states were persistent by race and economic status. [36] Figure 11.2 shows these state by state comparisons.

FIGURE 11.2

OVERALL STATE HEALTH SYSTEM PERFORMANCE:
Scorecard Ranking, 2017

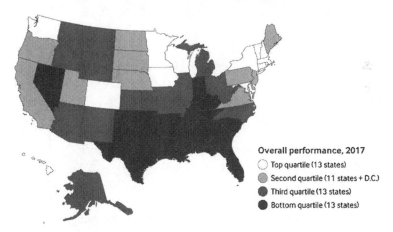

Source: D. C. Radley, D. McCarthy, and S. L. Hayes, *Aiming Higher: Results from the Commonwealth Fund Scorecard on State Health System Performance 2017 Edition*, The Commonwealth Fund, March 2017.

Source: D. C. Radley, D. McCarthy, and S. L. Hayes, *Aiming Higher: Results from the Commonwealth Scorecard on State Health System Performance* 2017 Edition, The Commonwealth Fund, March 2017.

- Periodic cross-national studies of 11 advanced countries conducted by the Commonwealth Fund find the U. S. remains the worst of these countries in terms of quality of care as measured by mortality amenable to health care, almost double that of France. [37] (Figure 11.3)

FIGURE 11.3

OVERALL STATE HEALTH SYSTEM PERFORMANCE: U.S. LAGS OTHER COUNTRIES: MORTALITY AMENABLE TO HEALTH CARE

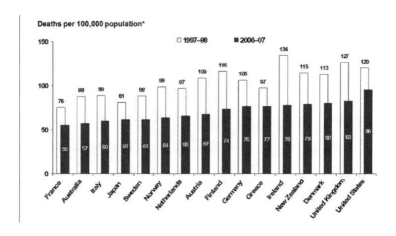

Lessons from failure to improve quality

These lessons seem inescapable given the lack of progress in improving the quality of U. S. health care over many years, despite some improvements in access brought by the ACA.

1. Financial barriers to care are increasing.
2. Uninsurance and underinsurance are increasing.
3. Socioeconomic determinants, racial and ethnic disparities leave millions of Americans without necessary health care.
4. Employed physicians today have less clinical autonomy and are pressured by their employers to over utilize services.

5. The shortage of primary care physicians leads to fragmentation and inadequate coordination of care that compromises quality of care.

6. Quality measures are flawed and don't represent what happens to patients.

7. FDA reviews for efficacy of drugs and medical devices need to be more rigorous and separated from political influences.

8. Medicare and Medicaid cuts threatened by GOP policies will lead to a more fragile safety net further compromising access and quality of care.

9. There is a lack of public accountability throughout our largely for-profit market-based system.

Given these lessons, the magnitude of fundamental health care reform becomes more clear. This recommendation by Dr. Donald Berwick, former administrator of CMS and president/CEO of the Institute for Healthcare Improvement, and two colleagues gives us an effective way forward to improving U. S. health care:

Improving the U. S. health care system requires simultaneous pursuit of three aims: improving the experience of care, improving the health of populations, and reducing per capita costs of health care. Preconditions for this include the enrollment of an identified population, a commitment to universality for its members, and the existence of an organization (an "integrator") that accepts responsibility for all three aims for that population. The integrator's role includes at least five components: partnership with individuals and families, redesign of primary care, population health management, financial management, and macro system integration. [38]

Concluding comment

Our increasingly privatized, corporatized market-based system is killing us. People are literally dying by the tens of thousands because of the lack of adequate health insurance, growing financial barriers to care, and persistent disparities by race and economic status. Our unaccountable market-based "system" is completely unsustainable. Just looking at the Medicaid budget gives us a strong reason to reform our financing system—sooner than later. Lawrence Brown, professor of health policy and management at Columbia University, warns us about the downsides of privatized health care:

> *No other nation expects a private sector, little constrained by public rules on the size and terms of employer contributions, to carry so heavy a burden of coverage and none asks private insurers to hold the line with providers (including specialists, uncommonly abundant in the United States) on prices outside a framework of public policies that guide the bargaining game. The first of these two grand exceptions largely accounts for the nation's high rates of un- and underinsurance; the latter mainly explains why America's health spending is so high by cross-national standards.* [39]

As we will see in Chapter 15, there is a fix that will save everyone money—patients, families, government at all levels—and at the same time extend necessary health care to all Americans. But for now, we'll turn to the next chapter to see how much our growing health care bureaucracy, mostly private, together with corruption and fraud, are wasting money that should be going to health care.

References:

1. U. S. Department of Commerce, Washington, D.C.
2. Pitt, WR. A lesson from my hospital bed: For-profit health care is a merciless sham. *Truthout*, June 21, 2017.
3. Siegel, R, Columbus, C. As cost of U. S. health care skyrockets, so does pay of health care CEOs. *NPR*, July 26, 2017.
4. Scully, T. As quoted by Davidson, A. The President wants you to get rich on Obamacare. *New York Times Magazine*, October 13, 2013.
5. Murphy, T. Aetna trumps 2Q expectations after scaling back ACA coverage. *ABC News*, August 3, 2017.
6. Milbank, D. Trump just told the truth. He may wish he hadn't. *The Washington Post*, December 20, 2017.
7. Potter, W. Health insurers working the system to pad their profits. Center for Public Integrity, August 15, 2015.
8. Livingston, S. With no fix in omnibus budget bill, insurers set to hike premiums, rethink selling individual plans. *Modern Healthcare*, March 23, 2018.
9. The high cost of healthcare: Patients see greater cost-shifting and reduced coverage in exchange markets 2014-2018. Physicians for Fair Coverage. Research by *Avalere*, July 2018.
10. Individual markets nationally face high premium increases in coming years absent federal or state action. *Covered California*, March 12, 2018.
11. Schulte, F. As seniors get sicker, they're more likely to drop Medicare Advantage plans. *Kaiser Health News*, July 6, 2017.
12. Schulte, F. Audits of some Medicare Advantage plans reveal pervasive overcharging. *NPR Now KPLU*, August 29, 2016.
13. Abelson, R. With mergers, concerns grow about private Medicare. *New York Times*, August 25, 2015.
14. Terhune, C, Gorman, A. Enriched by the poor: California health insurers make billions through Medicaid. *Kaiser Health News*, November 6, 2017.
15. Herman, B. Medicaid's unmanaged managed care. *Modern Healthcare*, April 30, 2016.

16. Himmelstein, DU, Woolhandler, S. The post-launch problem: the Affordable Care Act's persistently high administrative costs. *Health Affairs Blog*, May 27, 2015.

17. Kahn, CN. Intolerable risk, irreparable harm: The legacy of physician-owned hospitals. *Health Affairs (Millwood)* 25 (1): 130-133, 2006.

18. Bach, PB. Paying doctors to ignore patients. *New York Times*, July 24, 2008.

19. Olinger, D. Confusion about free-standing ER brings Colorado mom $5,000 bill. *The Denver Post*, October 31, 2015.

20. Phelan, M. *Social Security Works*, August 5, 2017.

21. Bever, L. A town of 3,200 was flooded with nearly 21 million pain pills as addiction crisis worsened, lawmakers say. *The Washington Post*, January 31, 2018.

22. Higham, S, Bernstein, L. The drug industry's triumph over the DEA. *The Washington Post*, October 15, 2017.

23. Harrington, C, Olney, B, Carrillo, H et al. Nurse staffing and deficiencies in the largest for-profit nursing home chains owned by private equity companies. *Health Serv Res* 47 (1): 106-128, 2012.

24. Cabin, W, Himmelstein, DU, Siman, ML et al. For-profit Medicare home health agencies' costs appear higher and quality appears lower compared to not-for-profit agencies. *Health Affairs* 33(8): 1460-1465, 2014.

25. Kutsher, B. Coverage parity draws investors to behavioral health. *Modern Healthcare*, July 20, 2015.

26. Cummings, JR, Wen, H, Ko, M. Decline in public substance abuse disorder treatment centers most serious in counties with high shares of black residents. *Health Affairs*, June 2016.

27. Whoriskey, P, Keating, D. Dying and profits: The evolution of hospice. *The Washington Post*, December 26, 2014.

28. Casalino, LP, Gans, D, Weber, R et al. U. S. physician practices spend more than $15.4 billion annually to report quality measures. *Health Affairs* 35: 401-406, 2016.

29. Seidman, J, Feore, J, Rosacker, N. Medicare accountable care organizations have increased federal spending contrary to projections that they would produce net savings. *Avalere*, March 29, 2018.

30. Maddox, KJ. As quoted by Rubin, R. How value-based Medicare payments exacerbate health care disparities. *JAMA*, February 21, 2018.

31. Patashnik, E. Why American doctors keep doing expensive procedures that don't work. *VOX*, February 14, 2018.

32. Bakalar, N. Medical errors may cause over 250,000 deaths a year. *New York Times*, May 3, 2016.

33. Beck, M. Wrong-patient errors called common. *Wall Street Journal*, September 26, 2016.

34. CDC reports 45,000 die each year for lack of health insurance. *Daily Kos*, October 15, 2012.

35. Healy, M. Doctors group calls on pediatricians to address child poverty. *Los Angeles Times*, March 9, 2016.

36. Radley, DC, McCarthy, D, Hayes, SL. Aiming Higher: Results from the Commonwealth Fund Scorecard on State Health System Performance. New York. *Commonwealth Fund*, 2017.

37. Osborn, R, Moulds, D. *The Commonwealth Fund 2014 International Health Policy Survey of Older Adults in Eleven Countries*, November 2014, p. 20.

38. Berwick, DM, Nolan, TW, Whittington, J. The triple aim: Care, health, and cost. *Health Affairs* 27 (3), May-June 2008.

39. Brown, LD. In Stevens, RA, Rosenberg, CE, Burns, LR (eds) *History and Health Policy in the United States: Putting the Past Back In*. New Brunswick, NJ. *Rutgers University Press*, 2006, p. 46.

CHAPTER 12

INCREASED BUREAUCRACY, WASTE, CORRUPTION, AND FRAUD

The U. S. health care system is by far the most bureaucratic and expensive system in the world, in large part because we have such an inefficient and profit-driven multi-payer financing system. In this chapter, we will describe the extent of increasing bureaucracy, waste, corruption and fraud that collectively decrease the monies available for direct patient care.

Increasing Bureaucracy

We cannot look to history for any guidance to address the problems of increasing bureaucracy in U. S. health care. The growth of managed care in the late 1980s and 1990s led to new oversized administrative bureaucracies as HMOs were marketed as new investor-owned for-profit companies. An ever-larger administrative bureaucracy was needed to set limits on referrals and hospitalizations, denial of services, disenrollment of sick enrollees, and such abuses as hiding performance data. [1] Between 2000 and 2005, when the insurance market declined by one percent, its workforce grew by one-third. [2] The ACA increased bureaucracy further as the exchanges became consumed with such activities as determining eligibility for qualified health plans and subsidies/tax credits and verifying annual household income and family size, which are subject to change from year to year. [3]

The chaos of TrumpCare insurance markets, both private and public, are making the bureaucracy of health care even worse. With all the changes under the Trump administration, patients' insurance status is more volatile than ever before. Just looking at privatized Medicaid shows us what a jungle the bureaucracy has become. As one example, imagine trying to implement work requirements in the states that adopt them. Even when many thousands of Medicaid beneficiaries gain work, many of their jobs will be hourly or temporary and subject to change month by month. Beyond the bureaucratic nightmare of administration, the required work policy is destined for failure on many counts. For example, many Medicaid beneficiaries cannot work for such reasons as illness, disability, unstable hours, caring for parents or children, and lack of available jobs in their area. [4] Sara Rosenbaum, health policy expert at George Washington University, makes this cogent observation:

People on Medicaid lead very hard lives. Seema Verma (CMS director) wants to make it harder. She doesn't seem to understand Medicaid as a public health system. Yet, she is breaking with more than 50 years of long-standing policy. [5]

As a result of this continued growth of bureaucracy in U. S. health care over these many years, physicians and their staffs are confronted with a huge time and energy burden every day that detracts from patient care and leads to increasing rates of physician burnout, especially in the more time-intensive specialties of primary care, geriatrics, and psychiatry. These are just some of the things they have to deal with before patients can be seen and treated for a primary care visit: insurance verification, pre-authorization for planned tests and procedures; determination of whether drugs will be covered by differing drug formularies among insurers; and arranging for specialist consultants after finding out their status in or out of network.

Agreements between health plans and participating physicians generally include a statement that the insurer has the right to determine the medical necessity of surgery, imaging studies, medication, and many other procedures. A recent poll by the American Medical Association concerning physician attitudes toward prior authorization (PA) found that 92 percent of respondents believe that it can have a negative impact on patient outcomes and that 84 percent find it to be a high or extremely high burden. The average time spent each week for prior authorization by physicians and their staffs was reported as 14.6 hours, or about two business days. [6] Dr. Halee Fischer-Wright, President and CEO of the Medical Group Management Association, brings us this important observation:

> *Health plan demands for approval for physician-ordered medical tests, clinical procedures, medications, and medical devices ceaselessly question the judgment of physicians, resulting in less time to treat patients and needlessly driving up administrative costs for medical groups.* [7]

Administrative costs of health care in this country have increased by more than 10 percent a year since 1971, and now account for more than 4 percent of our GDP. The dramatic growth in the numbers of administrators compared to physicians in the U. S. since 1970 bears witness to this unparalleled growth in health care bureaucracy. (Figure 12.1)

FIGURE 12.1

GROWTH OF PHYSICIANS AND ADMINISTRATORS - 1970-2017

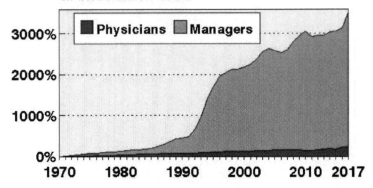

Growth Since 1970

Source: Bureau of Labor Statistics; NCHS; and Himmelstein/Woolhandler analysis of CPS.
Note - Managers shown as moving average of current year and 2 previous years

Waste

The growing costs of private insurance overhead and administration of insurers, physicians and other health care professionals takes both time and resources away from the main goal of the health care system—care of the patient. The overhead of the private health insurance industry now amounts to $792 per capita per year, more than five times that of Canada with its public single-payer financing system. Hospital administrative costs in the U. S. make up more than 25 percent of total hospital expenditures. Administrators in various other parts of the health care system have grown by 3,000 percent since 1970. Nurses in this country spend more than 13 hours each week to obtain prior authorizations for services, compared to none in Canada. [8]

Administrative costs are estimated to represent 25 to 31 percent of total health care expenditures in this country, twice that in Canada and considerably greater than in other OECD countries where these costs have been studied. At least 62 percent of these are for billing transactions. A recent analysis of the costs to process physician billings for professional services per patient encounter in the following settings found these results:

- Primary care visit: 13 minutes and $20.49
- Discharged Emergency Department visit: 32 minutes and $64.54
- General inpatient stay: 73 minutes and $124.26
- Ambulatory surgical procedure: 75 minutes and $170.40
- Inpatient surgical procedure: 100 minutes and $215.10 [9]

That study estimated that the costs of billing activities performed by primary care physicians translated to more than $99,000 per year for each primary care physician! It further estimated that the process of moving money from hospitals and physicians in the U. S. consumes some $500 billion per year, with about 80 percent of that being wasteful, including high rates of remittances that are three times higher than in other industries. [10]. CMS projects that more than $2.7 *trillion* will be spent for private health insurance overhead and administration of government health programs (mostly Medicare and Medicaid) between 2014 and 2022.

Administrative overhead of privatized Medicaid has gone through the roof, accounting for 22.5 percent of the federal government's total expenditures for the program, more than 11 times the administrative overhead of traditional, non-privatized Medicare.[11] How can privatized Medicare and Medicaid be justified to taxpayers when the costs of privatization are so high and wasteful?

Corruption

Donald Trump's promise as a presidential candidate that, if elected, he would "drain the swamp" of corruption and influence peddling has proven to be just another Trump lie. Instead, his administration has been stained by unprecedented conflicts of interest that start at the top. Despite the admonitions of ethicists and the U. S. Office of Government Ethics, he has refused to divest himself from his financial interests in his hotels, golf courses, restaurants, and real estate developments around the world. He has just said that he would "isolate" himself from the management of the Trump Organization and put his sons in charge of the operation of the worldwide company. His businesses were reshuffled into holding companies held by a trust that Trump controls himself. As Robert Weissman, president of Public Citizen, states:

> *Donald Trump entered office with the most blatant and potentially corrupting conflicts of interest in the history of American politics, and things got worse from there. Business is booming at Trump International Hotel in Washington, D.C. and other Trump properties not because of the décor, but because corporations and foreign governments want to curry favor with the president.* [12]

Unabashed by his hypocrisy over ethical standards, Trump signed Executive Order 13770 one week after his inauguration titled "Ethics Commitments by Executive Branch Appointees," supposedly intended to end the revolving door between K Street and the government, including an injunction against foreign lobbying. But just six months later, the liberal super PAC found 74 lobbyists working in the administration, 49 of them in agencies they once lobbied on behalf of clients. [13] Hui Chen, former federal prosecutor who was hired as a full-time compliance expert in the Justice Department's Fraud Section in 2015, resigned six months into the Trump administration with this parting statement:

> *Trying to hold companies to standards that our current administration is not living up to was creating a cognitive dissonance that I could not overcome. . . . I am not willing to compartmentalize my values as an [ethics and compliance] professional, a citizen, and a human being. . . . I wanted no more part [in an administration] that has so casually flouted ethics guidelines.* [14]

Despite the Executive Order, conflicts of interest and revolving door problems are pervasive in the thinly staffed Trump administration still marked by rapid turnover and ethical transgressions. Here are just four of many examples of today's toxic ethical climate in this administration.

- Fifteen months into his presidency, Trump spent more than 100 days at his own resorts/golf courses, mostly at Mar-a-Lago in Florida to wine and dine with his elitist club members and government dignitaries, at a cost of about $3.5 million per weekend trip. Taxpayers pay the bills for lodging and meals of Trump's staff and Secret Service detail while all profits go to Trump as owner of the resorts. [15]

- Despite his Executive Order, Trump has issued many waivers of those ethical standards, usually to individuals who had been retained by for-profit clients and then took up matters that could benefit these former clients. Larry Leggitt is one of many who received ethical waivers. He took in $400,000 as a lobbyist trying to influence

Medicare policy in 2016, later becoming chief of staff in the Department of Health and Human Services in the Trump administration. [16] Two of his registered lobbying clients in 2016 were the Arthroscopy Association of North America and Arriva Medical, a large supplier of diabetes testing products that has since closed down. [17]

- As Trump's first appointee to head the Department of Health and Human Services, Dr. Tom Price called for deep spending and staffing cuts in this department, including a $6 billion cut for the National Institutes of Health budget.[18]

- Mick Mulvaney, director of Office of Management and Budget, acknowledges that he has a hierarchy of whom he will talk to in a "pay to play" operation, with willingness to see lobbyists who have given him campaign donations but not those who did not. [19]

Fraud

Fraud in U. S. health care has long been a problem. Medical billing fraud, ironically enabled by electronic health records, is estimated to account for 10 percent of all health care costs, or about $270 billion a year. [20] There are many ways how hospitals and other providers can defraud the billing process, such as disguising claims, misrepresenting operating expenses, double billing, and submitting false claims for unnecessary services or those never received by patients. Managed care plans can falsify records, collude bid-rigging, charge exorbitant "administrative fees", and withhold payments to providers or subcontractors. All this is very complicated and beyond comprehension for most of us.

Malcolm Sparrow, Professor of the Practice of Public Management at Harvard's John F. Kennedy School of Government, with ten years' experience as a detective with the British police service earlier in his career, is the leading expert in this country on health care fraud. His 1996 book, updated in 2000, *License to Steal: How Fraud Bleeds America's Health Care System*, is still the classic in the field. In 2009, Professor Sparrow gave this sobering testimony before the Subcommittee on Crime and Drugs of the Senate Committee on the Judiciary:

> *The health industry's controls are weakest with respect to outright criminal fraud. By contrast the industry's controls perform reasonably well in managing the grey and more ambiguous issues, such as questions about medical orthodoxy, pricing, and the limits of policy coverage. But criminals, who are intent on stealing as much as they can as fast as possible, and who are prepared to fabricate diagnoses, treatments, even entire medical episodes, have a relatively easy time breaking through the industry's defenses. The criminals' advantage is that they are willing to lie. And provided they learn to submit their bills correctly, they remain free to lie. The rule for criminals is simple: if you want to steal from Medicare or Medicaid, or any other health care insurance program, learn to bill your lies correctly. Then, for the most part, your claims will be paid in full and on time, without a hiccup, by a computer, and with no human involvement at all.* [21]

The following examples throughout our health care system show how pervasive fraud continues as a major problem at the expense of patients, families, and taxpayers. Unfortunately, we can expect this problem to get worse the more privatization and deregulation of health care are pursued by the Trump administration.

- Federal audits of 37 private Medicare Advantage programs have revealed overspending due to inflated risk scores that overstated the severity of such conditions as diabetes and depression for a majority of elderly patients treated. [22]

- A recent investigation by the Office of Inspector General of DHHS found widespread fraud and abuse in the Personal Care Services program of privatized Medicaid plans. [23]

- Overpayments to privatized Medicaid plans are endemic in more than 30 states, often involving unnecessary or duplicative payments to providers. [24]

- Federal auditors have even found that private Medicaid insurers in Florida received $26 million over five years for coverage of dead people, mostly as a result of outdated information in state data bases and lack of coordination among different agencies. [25]

- Purdue Pharma, which gained FDA approval for OxyContin in 1995, hired 1,000 sales representatives to hype the drug's safety at medical conferences and physicians' offices, eventually generating some $35 billion in revenue. Purdue Pharma is owned by the Sackler family, which has a current net worth of $13 billion. Profit-driven corporate irresponsibility has contributed to the opioid crisis, as exemplified by two of the biggest drug distributors shipping more than 12 million doses of OxyContin to a single pharmacy in a tiny West Virginia town over an eight-year period. [26]

- Almost three-quarters of the more than 11,000 nursing homes in the country outsource a wide variety of goods and services to companies in which they control or have a financial interest; these "related party transactions" bring higher profits to nursing homes without being recorded in their financial records even as they cut nursing staff and put patients at increased risk. [27]

- A 13-year investigation by *The Washington Post* of for-profit hospices found the industry riddled with fraud and abuse, commonly seeking out less sick patients who need less care and live longer, yielding higher profits, and even encouraging their employees to recruit such patients. [28]

- Medical identity theft is on the rise whereby criminals steal personal data from millions of Americans to get health care, prescriptions and medical equipment; this can result in victims having claims denied, losing insurance coverage, and/or adverse impacts on their credit ratings. [29]

This is how Ralph Nader sums up the economic and political challenges in dealing with health care fraud:

All in all, the health care industry is replete with rackets that neither honest practitioners or regulators find worrisome enough to effectively challenge. The perverse economic incentives in this industry range from third party payments to third party procedures. Add paid-off members of Congress who starve enforcement budgets and the enormous profits that come from that tired triad 'waste, fraud and abuse' and you have a massive problem needing a massive solution. [30]

Concluding comment

There is a fix to what has become a long-term massive problem of escalating bureaucracy, waste, corruption and fraud driven by greed in an increasingly unaccountable system. Single-payer financing, with everyone having a Medicare for All card, would eliminate most of this, while saving more than $600 billion a year through simplified administration, negotiated fees for health professionals, global budgets for hospitals and other facilities, and transition toward a not-for-profit service oriented system. We will discuss all that in Chapter 15. But for now let's move to the next chapter where we will see that unaccountability of health care in the Trump administration is one more reason that today's health care policies will not work, are detrimental to the public interest, and are completely unsustainable.

References:

1. McCormick, D et al. Relationship between low quality-of-care scores and HMO's subsequent disclosure of quality-of-care scores. *JAMA* 288: 1484, 2002.

2. Krugman, P. The world of U. S. health care economics is downright scary. *Seattle Post Intelligencer*, September 26, 2006: B1.

3. Office of the Inspector General. Not all of the federally facilitated marketplace's internal controls were effective in ensuring that individuals were properly determined eligible for qualified health plans and insurance affordability programs. Department of Health and Human Services. Washington, D.C., August 2015.

4. Corcoran, M. Medicaid work requirements: Trump's war on the poor expands, one state at a time. *Truthout*, April 25, 2018.

5. Rosenbaum, S. As quoted by Corcoran, M. Ibid # 4.

6. AMA. 2017 AMA Prior Authorization Physician Survey, December 2017.

7. MGMA. Payer prior authorization requirements on physicians continue rapid escalation: increasing practice overhead and delaying patient care. Poll, May 16, 2017.

8. Geyman, JP. *Common Sense about Health Care Reform in America*. Friday Harbor, WA. *Copernicus Healthcare*, 2017, p. 12.

9. Tseng, P, Kaplan, RS, Richman, JD et al. Administrative costs associated with physician billing and insurance-related activities at an academic health care system. *JAMA*, February 20, 2018.

10. Ibid # 9.

11. Himmelstein, DU, Woolhandler, S. The post-launch problem: The Affordable Care Act's persistently high administrative costs. *Health Affairs Blog*, May 27, 2015.

12. Weisman, R, as quoted by Zibel, A. Presidency for sale. *Public Citizen News*, March/April 2018, pp. 8-9.

13. Nazaryan, A. The swamp runneth over. *Newsweek*, November 10, 2017.

14. Johnson, J. Top ethics official resigns, says working for Trump requires 'abandonment of conscience.' *Common Dreams*, July 3, 2017.

15. Rmuse, Opinion: Swindler Trump is using the White House to rip off taxpayers. *PoliticusUSA*, March 21, 2017.

16. Lipton, E, Ivory, D. Lobbyists, industry lawyers were granted ethics waivers to work in Trump Administration. *New York Times*, June 8, 2017.

17. Ackley, K. Trump administration gives ethics waivers to ex-lobbyists. *Roll Call*, June 7, 2017.

18. Finnegan, M, Barabak, MZ. Mnuchin, Price and others on Trump's team are getting taxpayer-funded travel perks—but where's the outrage? *Los Angeles Times*, September 26, 2017.

19. Markay, L, Stein, S. Mick Mulvaney met with lobbyist donors while at Trump White House. *Daily Beast*, April 27, 2018.

20. Buchheit, P. Private health care as an act of terrorism. *Common Dreams*, July 20, 2015: 1.

21. Sparrow, MK. Testimony before Senate Committee on the Judiciary, Subcommittee on Crime and Drugs. *Criminal Prosecution as a Deterrent to Health Care Fraud.* May 20, 2009.

22. Schulte, F. Audits of some Medicare Advantage plans reveal pervasive overcharging. *NPR Now* KPLU, August 29, 2016.

23. Bailey, M. Seniors suffer amid widespread fraud by Medicaid caretakers. *Kaiser Health News*, November 7, 2016.

24. Herman, B. Medicaid's unmanaged managed care. *Modern Healthcare*, April 30, 2016.

25. Chang, D. Florida paid Medicaid insurers $26 million to cover dead people, report says. *Miami Herald*, December 13, 2016.

26. Pizzigati, S. The Big PhRMA family that brought us the opioid crisis. *Common Dreams*, February 22, 2018.

27. Rau, J. Care suffers as more nursing homes feed money into corporate webs. *Kaiser Health News*, December 31, 2017.

28. McCauley, L. Investigation reveals rampant fraud by privatized hospice groups. *Common Dreams*, December 17, 2013.

29. Armour, S. The doctor bill from identity thieves. *Wall Street Journal*, August 8, 2015.

30. Nader, R. In the public interest. Follow the hospital bills. *The Progressive Populist* 18 (4): 19, March 1, 2012.

CHAPTER 13

INADEQUATE OVERSIGHT AND ACCOUNTABILITY

So it is that contrary to what we have heard rhetorically for a generation now, the individualist, greed-driven, free-market ideology is at odds with our history and with what most Americans really care about. More and more people agree that growing inequality is bad for the country, that corporations have too much power, that money in politics is corrupting democracy and that working families and poor communities need and deserve help when the market system fails to generate shared prosperity. Indeed, the American public is committed to a set of values that almost perfectly contradicts the conservative agenda that has dominated politics for a generation now.

—Bill Moyers, leading journalist, political commentator, and Television Hall of Famer [1]

The last five chapters have described how TrumpCare is bound to fail the public interest and common good while benefitting corporate stakeholders at the expense of everyday Americans. We have already seen how privatization and deregulation in our market-based system go hand in hand and do not assure access to affordable health care of acceptable quality. This chapter adds one more reason for TrumpCare's inevitable failure—the increasingly inadequate mechanisms for oversight and accountability of health care. This has been recognized by Bill Moyers as a long-term problem, but it is all the worse under the Trump administration.

This chapter has two goals: (1) to give examples that illustrate how the lack of oversight and accountability of health care is so widespread across our system; and (2) to discuss the necessary and appropriate role of government in ensuring adequate quality and safety of health care in this country.

Deteriorating Accountability under TrumpCare
Lower FDA standards

The Federal Drug Administration (FDA) dates back more than 100 years. It has an enormous job, bearing responsibility for the safety and efficacy of all human and veterinary drugs, biologic products, medical devices, and products emitting radiation that are sold in the U. S. User fees from the drug industry that it regulates make up a large part of its budget, so that the FDA is to a considerable extent held hostage by that industry. As a result, there are many ongoing conflicts of interest in its advisory committees and other parts of the approval process.

As it pushes for faster approval of its drugs on weaker evidence, the drug industry has successfully opposed the use of cost-effectiveness as a criterion for drug or device approval or requiring new drug applications to demonstrate benefit over competitor drugs, not just placebo. The FDA increasingly approves new drugs based on lower standards of evidence, then requires post-approval studies to further assess safety and efficacy. According to a recent study, however, only 54 percent of the mandated studies had been completed five or six years after approval and only 20 percent had even been studied. [2]

Unfortunately, the FDA is typically underfunded and lacks regulatory teeth.

Pharmaceutical industry

As we saw in Chapter 2 (page 39), the drug industry has effectively lobbied the government for many years to retain its ability to set drug prices and avoid price controls. Drug manufacturers set prices to whatever the market will bear as they lobby government to spread its influence in Washington, D. C. As just one example, Novo Nordisk, which produces Levemir, a long-acting insulin, runs its own political action committee (PAC) and has asked more than 400 of its employees to contact lawmakers and their staffs on Capitol Hill. It raised the wholesale price of a vial of Levimir from $144.80 in 2012 to $335.70 in 2018, and is under investigation by state attorneys general for predatory pricing. [3]

Meanwhile, of course, drug prices keep going up. Over the five years since 2013, prices for the top 20 drugs prescribed for older Americans rose by an average of 12 percent a year, with seven of those drugs increasing by more than 100 percent. [4]

Drug Enforcement Agency (DEA) and opioids

The use of *prescribed* opioids, such as hydrocodone and oxycodone, has soared over the last 20 years, led by a multi-faceted campaign underwritten by the pharmaceutical industry that touted the use of these drugs for chronic pain with little chance of addiction. Now we have an epidemic that has killed more than 200,000 Americans, more than three times the number of U. S. military deaths in the Vietnam War. Initially, Joe Rannazzisi of the DEA stood tall in enforcement actions against wholesale drug distributors that were shipping huge volumes of prescription opioids to targeted corrupt physicians and pharmacists engaged in a very lucrative black market.

A powerful backlash from industry, however, soon began to neutralize the DEA through recruitment by the pharmaceutical industry of at least 56 DEA and DOJ officials and PAC committees calling for legislative action. Spearheaded by Rep. Tom Marino (R-PA), the result was the passage of the disingenuously named Ensuring Patient Access and Effective Drug Enforcement Act of 2016 that raised the bar for enforcement to a "higher standard", from "an imminent danger to the community" to "a substantial likelihood of an imminent threat." That law made it almost impossible for the DEA to freeze suspicious shipments of hundreds of millions of opioid pills from wholesalers, and the number of enforcement actions by the DEA dropped precipitously. Rannazzisi was forced out of the DEA in 2015, then Trump nominated Marino to head up the Office of National Drug Control Policy until his name was withdrawn after his role in defanging the DEA was exposed by an investigative report by *The Washington Post* and *CBS 60 Minutes*. [5] Today, lawsuits have been filed in federal court in five states bringing claims of fraud and racketeering as well as unjust profits made by defendant companies. [6]

Private insurers

The Trump administration is promoting short-term insurance plans that offer lower premiums, "more choice", and much less coverage in getting around the ACA's requirement to cover ten essential benefits. The big tradeoff is lower premiums for less protection for healthy people, to the extent that these plans hardly qualify as insurance. A recent study by the Kaiser Family Foundation of short-term policies in 45 states plus the District of Columbia found that none covered maternity care, 71 percent excluded outpatient prescription drugs, 62 percent do not cover substance abuse disorders, and 43 percent don't cover mental health services. The cheapest plans have very high deductibles and other cost sharing exceeding $20,000. [7]

Short-term plans will exacerbate two public health crises—the worst rate of maternal deaths in the developed world and the deadliest drug epidemic in U. S. history. They also destabilize the risk pool for health insurance, attracting healthier people, avoiding those with such "deniable" conditions as diabetes, cancer, pregnancy, or HIV/AIDS, and raising premiums for older, sicker people to an unaffordable extent. More insurers are complaining of shrinking markets and a "death spiral" for the private health insurance industry.

Privatized Medicare and Medicaid

As we saw in Chapter 5 (pages 83-84), privatization of both of these essential programs leads to gaming the reimbursement system for higher profits, long waiting times, worse care, and often fraud. As a result, taxpayers and the government pay more and get less with little oversight or accountability.

Payment abuses

Today's reimbursement system with multiple payers has led to widespread abuses in payments to physicians and other health professionals. California gives us insight into what is going on. Despite passage of a state law in 2000 intended to rein in payment abuses by health care service plans, a recent survey reported these findings:

- Two-thirds of physician respondents had routine problems with unfair payment practices, such as repeated delays in adjudication and correct reimbursement of their claims.
- More than one-half of the physician practices reported that health plans attempted to rescind or modify authorizations after physicians had provided the services in good faith.
- Resolution processes were largely ineffective.
- Anthem and Blue Shield of California had the most unfair payment practices.

- Statewide, the Department of Managed Health Care has taken few enforcement actions against plans that engage in unfair payment practices. [8]

Nursing homes

Nursing homes across the country have serious safety and accountability problems. Infection control is routinely ignored. At the same time, the Trump administration has scaled back the use of penalties to punish nursing homes that violate standards that put residents at risk of injury. Part of the problem is the practice of three-quarters of U. S. nursing homes, in their pursuit of higher profits, to outsource services to companies that they control or in which they have an interest. Commonly owned companies are more likely to engage in and conceal fraud while having higher rates of patient injury than their not-for-profit counterparts. [9] Discharges and evictions have become a top-ranking category of grievances among nursing home residents, especially when their Medicare coverage reaches its limits. [10]

Assisted living

According to a 2018 report by the Government Accountability Office, many billions of dollars of government spending are going to deregulated assisted living facilities that operate under a patch-work of vague standards and limited oversight by state and federal authorities. The care of hundreds of thousands of patients, especially Medicaid beneficiaries, is jeopardized in these facilities, where elder abuse is widespread, including physical, emotional, and sexual abuse of residents. [11]

Prisons: non-payment of court fines and mental illness

As we saw in Chapter 5 (page 88), for-profit private prisons have become a huge industry that operates below the radar with little accountability. As Trump and Republican legislators were celebrating their December 2017 historic tax-cut (mostly for the wealthy), Trump's appointee as Attorney General reinstated a draconian policy that targets the poor—return to the equivalent of debtors' prisons. They were banned in the U. S. in 1833 and the Supreme Court has affirmed on three different occasions in the last century that the 14th Amendment prohibits incarceration for non-payment of exorbitant court-imposed fines or fees. Unfortunately, many cities have grown to rely on these fines and fees as a major source of revenue. [12]

Many more people with mental illness are housed across the U. S. in jails than in psychiatric hospitals. This is a major problem, since those in jails have poor access to psychiatric care. There tends to be insufficient staff training to deal with the mentally ill, to the extent that inmate suicides, self-mutilation and violence frequently result. [13]

Dismantling of the Environmental Protection Agency (EPA)

The EPA has been charged with safeguarding our air, water, land and climate from corporate polluters for almost 50 years. Scott Pruitt, as Trump's appointee to head the EPA, during his former six years as Oklahoma's Attorney General sued the EPA at least 14 times to block clean air and water standards, at the bidding of fossil fuel companies and other big polluters. As one example of Pruitt's attack on the EPA's original role, he granted a "financial hardship" waiver to billionaire investor Carl Icahn, who reported a net income of $234.4 million in 2017. [14] Robert Redford, longtime Board Member of the National Resources Defense Council (NRDC), sums up the serious concerns this way:

> *Administrator Pruitt is tearing down environmental safeguards while putting his agency at the beck and call of industries that exist to pollute and profit. You can be sure the*

rest of us will pay the price—in deadly smog, undrinkable water,
devastated wildlands, and a drastically warming climate. [15]

Although he has resigned, it appears that his successor will continue
these policies.

Role of Government in Ensuring Accountability of Health Care

It is time to admit that an unfettered market-based system with
little real competition and increasing consolidation by corporate
giants will never lead to a health care system that serves the common
good. Obama's ACA made some progress in expanding the number
of Americans with health insurance, but there are still more than 30
million uninsured, tens of millions underinsured, and cost containment
is nowhere in sight. This is how an overview assessment in *The
Lancet*, a leading medical journal in the U. K., sees our situation:

> *What Americans got with the Affordable Care Act was
> complicated insurance marketplaces in every state with a
> complex array of confusing private insurance products. The
> health reform process was exposed, in the words of the British
> medical journal The Lancet, "How corporate influence renders
> the U. S. government incapable of making policy on the basis of
> evidence and the public interest."* [16]

Dr. Marcia Angell, former editor of *The New England Journal
of Medicine* and author of *The Truth About Drug Companies: How
They Deceive Us and What We Can Do About It*, brings us this
important insight:

> *The fatal flaw in Obamacare is that it is inherently unsus-
> tainable. (Unfortunately, the Republicans are right that it is un-
> raveling, but wrong about the reason, and certainly wrong that*

the solution is more market competition.) Obama made the mistake of trying to increase access to better health insurance without fundamentally altering the features of our health system that made it so expensive, inflationary, and inadequate in the first place. Thus he continued to rely on investor-owned insurance companies and even guaranteed them millions more customers, while he also relied on revenue-seeking providers, including hospital conglomerates (even if technically nonprofit), out-patient facilities, drug companies, and medical specialists paid to provide ever more and ever pricier tests and procedures. . . . The result is that we still don't have a health care system. Rather, we have a non-system, consisting of thousands of businesses operating more or less independently of one another, each seeking to expand revenues and profits, often by avoiding uninsured or otherwise costly patients. [17]

TrumpCare has made access to affordable health care progressively worse. Increasing privatization, further deregulation, and shifting responsibility for health care to the states all work to increase waste and bureaucracy as the nation's safety net unravels further. Our present health care policies fail the public interest and benefit corporate stakeholders at the expense of patients, their families, and taxpayers. The prognosis for our non-system is poor unless we can acknowledge failure of our present directions and adopt fundamental reforms to be described in Chapter 15. Otherwise we can expect budget cuts and federal waivers to states, uncontrolled health care prices, and growing numbers of preventable early deaths due to the high costs of drugs and the lack of insurance coverage.

If we are to improve and reform our system, we need more government involvement in health care instead of less. The following are areas where federal government oversight is critical, with health policy based on experience and evidence, protected from corporate influence and lobbyists.

1 Establish and protect universal access to affordable health care for all Americans through single-payer Medicare for All.

2. Price controls, including negotiated prices of drugs and medical devices.

3. Global budgets for hospitals and other facilities; negotiated fees for physicians and other health professionals.

4. Planning for new facilities based on population needs for adequate access.

5. Workforce planning, to include goals to rebuild shortage fields, especially in primary care, psychiatry, and geriatrics; revision of present graduation medical education financing policies to support these goals.

6. Strengthen the authority of such federal agencies as the FDA and DEA, including adequate funding and protection from political influence.

7. Establish a national agency for science-based evaluation of treatments, based on efficacy and cost-effectiveness, free from conflicts of interest with industry.

8. Adopt policies intended to limit health care disparities, support equity, and reinforce a service ethic in health care.

Concluding comment

You can't deregulate a failing health care system if you want to improve and reform it in the public interest. There are stark differences between TrumpCare and GOP health care proposals and needed reforms in the public interest. The results will be bad if

GOP policies are not blocked by progressive Democrats in coming election cycles. The next two years give us an opportunity to finally get health care reform right, as we will discuss in Chapter 17.

References:

1. Moyers, B. A new story for America. *The Nation* 284 (3):17, 2007.
2. Woloshin, S, Schwartz, LM, White, BA et al. The fate of FDA post-approval studies. *N Engl J Med* 377: 1114-1117, September 2017.
3. Hancock, J, Lucas, E. How a drug company under pressure for high prices ratchets up political activity. *Kaiser Health News*, April 30, 2018.
4. Wapner, J. Pharmapocalypse. *Newsweek.com*, May 4, 2018.
5. Geyman, JP. The opioid epidemic: fueled by greed, corruption, and complicit government. *Daily Kos* and others, October 19, 2017.
6. Randazzo, S. New front in opioid lawsuits: rise in insurance premiums. *Wall Street Journal*, May 3, 2018.
7. Pollitz, K. Yes, the Trump administration promotes consumer choice—for healthy people. *The Washington Post*, May 1, 2018.
8. California Medical Association. CMA survey finds rampant health plan payment abuses. April 2, 2018.
9. Gorman, A. Weak oversight blamed for poor care at California nursing homes going unchecked. *Kaiser Health News*, May 4, 2018.
10. Bernard, TS, Pear, R. Complaints about nursing home evictions rise, and regulators take note. *New York Times*, February 22, 2018.
11. Pear, R. U. S. pays billions for 'assisted living,' but what does it get? *New York Times*, February 3, 2018.
12. Tesfaye, S. A return to debtors' prisons: Jeff Sessions' war on the poor. *Truthout*, December 31, 2017.
13. Gorman, A. Use of psychiatric drugs soars in California jails. *Kaiser Health News*, May 8, 2018.
14. Conley, J. Federal probe demanded after Trump's billionaire pal Carl Icahn receives EPA waiver worth tens of millions. *Common Dreams*, April 30, 2018.

15. Redford, R. New York. *NRDC*, April, 2018.

16. Ansell, DA, *The Death Gap: How Inequality Kills.* Chicago and London. *University of Chicago Press*, 2017, p. 137; quoting *The Lancet* 374, December 5, 2009.

17. Angell, M. Single payer: the single path. *Democracy. A Journal of Ideas.* Winter 2017.

What Now? Just Two Options Ahead

The idea of a common good was once widely understood and accepted in America. After all, the U. S. Constitution was designed for 'We the people' seeking to 'promote the general welfare'—not for 'me the narcissist' seeking as much wealth and power as possible. . . . If we're losing our national identity it's not because we now come in more colors, practice more religions, and speak more languages than we once did. It is because we are forgetting the real meaning of America—the ideals on which our nation was built. We are losing our sense of the common good.

—Robert B. Reich, professor of public policy at the University of California Berkeley, chairman of Common Cause, and author of the new book, *The Common Good* [1]

Reference:

1. Reich, R. Has the real meaning of America been lost? *San Francisco Chronicle*, February 20, 2018.

CHAPTER 14

CURRENT CRISIS IN U. S. HEALTH CARE

Something inside the human spirit cries out against the injustice of inequality when you know people who have to choose between food and medicine in a country where CEOs make more in an hour than their lowest-paid employees make in a month.

—The Reverend Dr. Barber II, WJ, president of the North Carolina chapter of the NAACP, pastor at Greenleaf Christian Church in Goldsboro, North Carolina, and founder of Repairers of the Breach [1]

In previous chapters we examined how TrumpCare has sabotaged the ACA and led to a far more dysfunctional health care system that increasingly fails the needs of ordinary Americans. It is now time to review the current crisis and chaos that cries out for fundamental reform. The goals of this chapter are (1) to briefly consider some societal trends that have allowed these changes to occur; and (2) to summarize the critical failings of TrumpCare today.

Historical Context

We can better understand how our dysfunctional and unfair health care system has developed and persists, especially over the last 30 years, when we consider the historical context of these years. Steven Brill, author of *America's Bitter Pill: Money, Politics, Backroom Deals, and the Fight to Fix Our Broken Healthcare*

System (2015) and his most recent 2018 book, *Tailspin: The People and Forces Behind America's Fifty-Year Fall—and Those Fighting to Reverse It,* brings us this useful historical perspective:

- *The country is now split into two classes: the protected and unprotected. The protected overmatched, overran and paralyzed the government. The unprotected were left even further behind.*
- *Income inequality has soared: inflation-adjusted middle class wages have been nearly frozen for the last four decades, while earnings of the top 1% have nearly tripled.*
- *Although the U. S. remains the world's richest country, it has the third-highest poverty rate among the 35 nations in the OECD.*
- *Nearly one in five American children live in a household that the government classifies as "food insecure."*
- *Congress has not passed a comprehensive budget on time without omnibus bills since 1994, which become targets for the more than 20 registered lobbyists working to block anything that would tax, regulate or otherwise threaten a deep-pocketed client.*
- *CEOs of largest U. S. firms take in an average of $15 million per year, almost 300 times more than typical workers.*
- *[Today's robber barons] have invested their winnings not only to preserve their bounty, but also to root themselves and their offspring in a new meritocracy-aristocracy that is more entrenched than the old-boy network.* [2]

In their 2017 book, *One Nation After Trump: A Guide for the Perplexed, the Disillusioned, the Desperate, and the Not-Yet-Deported*, Dionne, Ornstein and Mann make this helpful observation:

Rolling back the Trump threat requires seeing that he represents an extreme acceleration of a process that was long underway. It involves the decline of basic norms in politics, governing, and the media as well as the decay of institutions that are central to republican government. The radicalization of the Republican Party and its primary electorate began three decades ago. Absent these forces, Trump would still be a loudmouthed developer and brand-peddler far removed from the levers of power. [3]

Our democracy is under attack, as illustrated by the ongoing war between fake and real news and the spread of propaganda from the Trump administration, including its attempts to weaken the judiciary and discredit the Mueller investigation. Harvard political scientists Steven Levitsky and Daniel Ziblatt have studied the breakdown of democracies in Europe and Latin America for 20 years. Here is what they have to say about where we are in the U. S. in their 2018 book, *How Democracies Die*:

Today the guardrails of American democracy are weakening. The erosion of our democratic norms began in the 1980s and 1990s and accelerated in the 2000s . . . Trump may have accelerated this process, but he didn't cause it. The challenges facing American democracy run deeper. The weakening of our democratic norms is rooted in extreme partisan polarization— one that extends beyond policy differences into an existential conflict over race and culture. [4]

There can be no question but that Americans are increasingly polarized even as they become more anxious and fearful of today's times and their future. Trump's nativist language and frequent bigoted comments have fueled this growing polarization under the

Make America Great rubric that foments the white supremacist movement. Referring to a working paper entitled "White Outgroup Intolerance and Declining Support for American Democracy," by political scientists Steven V. Miller of Clemson and Nicholas T. Davis of Texas A & M, Noah Berlatsky has recently commented that:

> *The main threat to our democracy may be the hardening of one political ideology. . . The growing concentration of intolerant white voters in the GOP has created a party which appears less and less committed to the democratic project. When faced with a choice between bigotry and democracy, too many Americans are embracing the first while abandoning the second.* [5]

Crises Throughout the System: A Summary

Growing crises are rampart across all parts of U. S. health care despite a prevailing meme held by many conservatives that we have the best health care in the world. Policies on health care by the Trump administration are exacerbating problems, as these examples make clear.

1. Inadequate Access

Having adequate health insurance is becoming more elusive under TrumpCare. There are 28 million Americans uninsured in 2018, with this number growing to 32 million in 2019 and 41 million in 2025, according to CBO estimates. [6] Tens of millions more will be underinsured, especially as the Trump administration promotes short-term plans of less than one year that have attractively low premiums but high deductibles and minimal coverage, hardly enough to be considered insurance. Most of these "cheap" short-term plans will exclude coverage of pre-existing conditions, preventive care, maternity care, mental health or substance abuse treatment, and pharmaceuticals. Some will have deductibles up to $10,000 and co-pays up to 50 percent. [7]

With the ending of CSR payments, the insurance marketplace has become further destabilized. In response, insurers are continuing to raise premiums way beyond the cost of living for "inclusive plans." As two examples in Maryland, CareFirst BlueCross BlueShield has requested a 91 percent increase on its PPO plans and Kaiser Permanente wants a 37 percent hike on its HMO plans. [8] Insurers are also exiting more markets, thereby increasingly segmenting risk pools to patients' disadvantage.

Trump's recently proposed rules for health insurance loosen insurance regulations, and call for expansion of association health plans. These proposals have been widely opposed by consumer advocates, physician and nurse organizations, and trade groups representing insurers, hospitals, and clinics across the country. [9]

When we look at specific parts of the system, the situation is dire, as these examples show.

- *Community health centers* are private, nonprofit organizations that provide primary care services to residents of a defined medically underserved area. They make up the largest primary care network for some 26 million people in underserved areas. A majority of their funding comes from the federal Community Health Center Fund, which has and continues to be on the chopping block by fiscal conservatives. [10]

- *Women's health care.* The Trump administration is remaking federal policy on women's reproductive health along ideologic lines that greatly restrict women's choices, all in the name of "pro life." Even though the numbers of births and abortions are at an all-time low, Trump's proposed rules would forbid federally funded family planning clinics from referring women for abortions.

They would also make big changes in Title X, the family planning program that serves 4 million low-income people, including banning clinics from sharing physical space and financial resources with abortion providers. GOP efforts to defund Planned Parenthood continue, although 97 percent of its services are for preventive services such as contraceptive options, breast exams and screening for cervical cancer and sexually transmitted infections with only 3 percent for abortion services. Other regulatory proposals would emphasize "natural family planning" and abstinence. [11] The ironies and hypocrisy of these proposed rules are well illustrated by these observations:

> *The strange thing about this is that people who want to decrease the number of abortions are taking away access to the very services that help prevent them.*
>
> —Dr. Hal Lawrence, CEO of the American College of Obstetricians and Gynecologists. [12]

> *I do not believe that just because you're opposed to abortion, that makes you pro-life. I think in many cases, your morality is deeply lacking if all you want is a child born but not fed, not a child educated, not a child housed. And why would I think that you don't? Because you don't want any tax money to go there. That's not pro-life. That's pro-birth. We need a much broader conversation on what the morality of pro-life is.*
>
> —Sister Joan D. Chittister, O.S.B., a social psychologist with a Ph.D. from Penn State University and author of the 2015 book, *Between the Dark and the Daylight.* [13]

- *Childrens' health care.* The Children's Health Insurance Program (CHIP) provides care for about 9 million children and 370,000 pregnant women nationwide. Trump's 2018 budget cut billions from CHIP over two years and limited eligibility for federal matching funds. Ongoing funding for this important program is in jeopardy and remains a political football between the states and the federal government. [14]

- *Mental health care.* Mental health disorders affect one in five adults in this country, and are the leading cause of disability. But mental health care is poorly covered by private insurers, and payment for psychiatric services is so low that many health professionals avoid care of these patients. [15] There is a critical shortage of state psychiatric beds across the country that forces severely mentally ill patients to be held in emergency rooms, hospitals and jails while they await for a bed, sometimes for weeks. [16]

2. Increasing disparities

Disparities are increasing for much of our population in our dysfunctional profit-oriented system, thereby placing a higher burden of illness, injury, disability and mortality experienced by one population group compared to another. These disparities can be based on such factors as race/ethnicity, socioeconomic status, age, location, gender and disability status. Figure 14.1 illustrates how race/ethnicity impacted access to care for different groups in 2014.[17] Disparities can vary widely from one state to another. In Alabama, for example, low-income adults are almost seven times more likely than high-income people to report skipping needed care because of cost. [18]

A recent study by researchers at the University of Washington of years of life lost among people between ages 20 and 50 years old found a marked increase in premature deaths due to alcohol, drugs, suicide, and interpersonal violence from 1990 to 2016. [19] Labeled by some as "deaths of despair," the researchers found a considerable variation from one state to another, with 21 states reporting *higher* numbers of these premature deaths over that time period. [20]

FIGURE 14.1

PERCENT OF NONELDERLY ADULTS WHO DID NOT RECEIVE OR DELAYED CARE IN THE PAST 12 MONTHS BY RACE/ETHNICITY, 2014

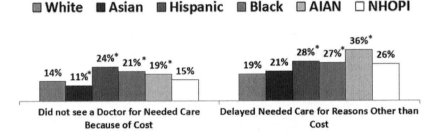

* Indicates statistically significant difference from the White population at the p<0.05 level. Note: AIAN refers to American Indians and Alaskan Natives. NHOPI refers to Native Hawaiians and Other Pacific Islanders. Persons of Hispanic origin may be of any race but are categorized as Hispanic for this analysis; other groups are non-Hispanic. Included nonelderly individuals of 18-64 years of age.

Source: Kaiser Family Foundation analysis of CDC,
Behavioral Risk Factor Surveillance System, 2014.

Dr. H. Jack Geiger, founding member and past president of Physicians for Human Rights and past president of Physicians for Social Responsibility, says this about these persistent health disparities:

> *What we deal with in our work, quite apart from the extremes of genocide, is a variant of that: "Lives less worthy of life." When we say that the poor have a mortality rate that is multiple times the rate of the rich, when we say poor children die in our country and in the developing world at rates far higher than*

those of the better off, we are saying that we permit a condition which in effect says that they are less worthy of life. We are sending this message because we let it happen, because we have social policies that almost assure that it will happen, and we let it happen stubbornly and continually. [21]

Despite the magnitude of these continuing disparities, there is evidence that they can be effectively addressed. A 2006 survey by the Commonwealth Fund found that many disparities in access and quality of care disappeared among blacks and Hispanics who had stable insurance and access to a high-performing primary care medical home. [22]

3. Unaffordable Costs of Care

The costs of health care in the U. S. have continued to rise exponentially with no end in sight. A large and growing part of the population cannot afford necessary health care. The 2018 Milliman Medical Index reports that the typical working American family of four covered by an average employer-sponsored preferred provider organization (PPO) now pays more than an average of $28,000 per year for health care, on insurance premiums, cost-sharing and forgone wage increases (for the employer contribution.)

The components of this spending on health care break down this way:

Inpatient: 31 percent ($8,631)

Outpatient: 19 percent ($5,395)

Professional services: 29 percent ($8,275)

Pharmacy: 17 percent ($4,888)

Other: (egs. home health, ambulance, prosthetics: 4 % ($995) [23]

The median annual household income in the U. S. is now $59,358 and the Commonwealth Fund defines financial hardship for health care above 10 percent of annual income. These costs are almost one-half of annual income and clearly far beyond the wallets of ordinary Americans.

The Kaiser Family Foundation tracks these numbers in terms of the "medical bill score." Their polls have found that 31 percent of Americans age 18 to 64 report that they or a family member face problems paying their health care bills; that number goes up to 57 percent if they are sick. As a result, 72 percent put off vacations or household purchases, 70 percent cut back on food, 59 percent used up all or most of their savings, and 41 percent took an extra job or worked more hours. [24]

Medical bills are a leading source of bankruptcy in the U. S. Even more commonly, medical debt exacts widespread damage to people's credit scores, with almost 40 percent of adults younger than 65 reporting lower credit scores for this reason. [25]

4. Inadequate Quality of Care

For those who think or assume that health care in this country is better than anywhere else, these sobering measures indicate the opposite: [26]

- There has been a 50 percent increase in deaths from suicide, alcohol, and drug use since 2005.
- In 2016, average life expectancy at birth in the U. S. declined for a second year in a row.
- After trending downward for most of the last decade, rates of premature death from preventable or treatable causes are going up.

- 39 percent of adults in Mississippi and West Virginia are obese; one-quarter are obese even in states with the lowest rates.
- Across states, 41 percent to 66 percent of adults with symptoms of a mental illness (some of whom may not have been diagnosed) received no treatment in 2013-2015.
- Up to one-third of children needing mental health care in 2016 did not receive it, according to their parents.
- 29 percent of adults with employer-based insurance receive unneeded lower back imaging at diagnosis.
- Despite having Medicare, U. S. seniors with multiple chronic conditions or functional limitations report high rates of emergency department use and care coordination failures. [27]
- The two-thirds of the nation's nursing homes dependent on Medicaid funding have lower staffing and worse quality of care than others. [28]
- Missed visits and neglect are common for patients on hospice dying at home. [29]

We have a health care divide in this country which has much to do with where we live and one's ability to access high-quality health care and live a healthy life. Figure 14.2 shows these stark differences between better-than-average states and worse-than-average states.

5. *Instability and Volatility*

Our incoherent health care non-system has never been more unstable as the roles of insurers, hospitals, clinics, and corporate stakeholders continue to change, mostly chasing larger market share and higher revenues. Here are just three examples of the changing health care landscape without much clarity for its future.

FIGURE 14.2

AMERICA'S HEALTH CARE DIVIDE
STATE HEALTH SYSTEM PERFORMANCE
VARIES ACROSS THE COUNTRY

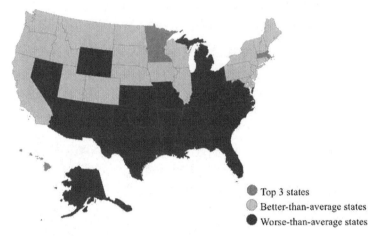

Top 3 states
Better-than-average states
Worse-than-average states

Source: 2018 Scorecard on State Health System Performance.
The Commonwealth Fund

- UnitedHealth, one of the largest private insurers, has purchased DeVita, a large for-profit chain of dialysis centers with almost 300 clinics [30]; before this purchase, UnitedHealth was already working with more than 30,000 physicians across 230 urgent care clinics and 200 surgery centers. [31]

- CVS Health, the second largest drugstore chain, has bought Aetna, the third largest insurer; this could lead to a network of clinics in almost 10,000 drugstores around the country. [32]

- Dignity Health and Catholic Health Initiatives plan to become a national chain of Catholic hospitals and clinics in 28 states with 139 hospitals and more than 25,000 physicians and other clinicians. [33]

Through these mergers, corporate stakeholders are trying to expand into new roles within a turbulent transformation of health care. No longer will physicians' offices be the hub of the system as urgent care centers and retail clinics proliferate in new locations, including drug stores and shopping malls. A battle is raging among competing interests for control of the primary care patient, which will determine where patients are hospitalized, where they fill their prescriptions, and where they receive laboratory tests and imaging procedures.

Patients are left out of this increasingly volatile system, with merging corporate stakeholders pursuing their own self-interest in a less accountable system rather than service to patients. Patients will likely see less choice of health care providers, higher costs, more fragmentation and less continuity of care. Meanwhile, they face churning of insurance coverage, which will become even worse if the GOP succeeds in cuts to Medicare and Medicaid. Some insurers are now even questioning the need for emergency room visits, thereby imposing large uncovered costs on patients for the follow-up care that results. [34]

6. Deteriorating Safety Net

Within all this turbulence in health care, the nation's safety net under the Trump administration is falling apart. These examples show how vulnerable lower-income Americans now struggle to survive in an increasingly cruel and uncaring society.

- 41 million Americans, larger than the combined populations of Texas, Michigan, and Maine, are classified by the U. S. Department of Agriculture as "food insecure." Family food insecurity exceeds 14 percent of those living in urban and rural areas. [35] The Supplemental Nutrition

Assistance Program (SNAP), commonly known as food stamps, was taken away from 2 million poor people as part of the May 2018 farm bill passed by Congress, even though it failed to save any money. [36] Food stamps also fail to cover the actual costs of a low-income meal in 99 percent of U. S. counties and the District of Columbia. [37]

- Subject to congressional approval, Trump wants to rescind $5 billion for the popular Children's Health Insurance Program (CHIP).After signing the March 2018 spending bill, the president has been pushed by conservatives in Congress to cut the federal deficit, which is projected to be almost $1 trillion in 2019. [38]

- Women are more likely than men to have low incomes and be the primary caretakers of their children. Since 40 million women are on Medicaid, they are especially vulnerable to cuts in safety net programs. Despite these facts, the Trump administration is disinvesting in women and families by such means as cuts in food stamps, reducing family planning funding, promoting short-term insurance policies without maternity coverage, imposing new work requirements for Medicaid, and proposals that would raise rents for low-income families. [39]

- About 7 million retirees who have depended on long-term care insurance are facing steep premium increases for less coverage. More than one-half of U. S. adults are expected to need nursing home or other care services. Long-term care typically costs at least $100,000 a year per individual. The long-term care insurance industry, however, is dying, with most insurers leaving this market. [40]

- Medicaid coverage, unstable at best and facing likely cutbacks at both federal and state levels, varies greatly from one state to another, as shown by Figure 14.3 [41] Nursing homes and group homes in Louisiana give us one current example of what these cuts can mean in one state. If proposed cuts are made, more than 30,000 Medicaid recipients will lose their benefits and face eviction.[42]

FIGURE 14.3

THE MEDICAID LANDSCAPE: STATE-BY-STATE COVERAGE

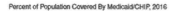
Percent of Population Covered By Medicaid/CHIP, 2016

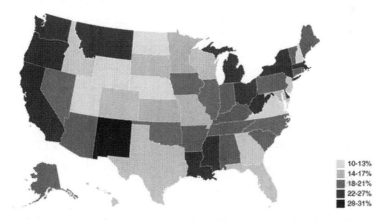

10-13%
14-17%
18-21%
22-27%
28-31%

Note: Includes those covered by Medicaid, the Children's Health Insurance Program (CHIP) and those who have both Medicaid and another type of coverage, such as dual eligibles who are also covered by Medicare.

Katrina vanden Heuvel, editor and publisher of *The Nation*, comments on this dire situation:

The administration is using the pretense of fiscal responsibility to slash programs for the poor and people of color. . . . When you have policies that take away the human rights of the poor and make women and children prey, then you have a nation that can't survive. [43]

The ugly underbelly of conservatives' attacks on welfare is exposed and fueled by Trump's racist rhetoric and the white supremacy movement to Make America Great. A recent study by two sociology researchers at the University of California Berkeley and Stanford University concludes that opposition to welfare has risen sharply among whites. Racial anxiety appears to be driving their calls for deeper cuts in welfare programs more than their conservative principles. [44]

Concluding comment

As a result of all this turmoil within health care, we have a rudderless, unaccountable "system" without a moral compass, aided and abetted by an enabling hands-off government. Patients and families are losing out as corporate giants vie for a bigger piece of the health care pie. Taxpayers can't afford this wasteful system at either the state or federal level. In today's polarized political climate, we have just two major options for reform—continue with TrumpCare as the sabotaged version of the ACA or support real reform through a single-payer Medicare for All system committed to the common good of all Americans. We will discuss those two alternatives in the next chapter.

References:

1.   Barber II, WJ. *The Third Reconstruction: How a Moral Movement Is Overcoming the Politics of Division and Fear*. Boston. *Beacon Press*, 2016, p. xiii.

2.   Brill, S. My generation was supposed to level America's playing field. Instead, we rigged it for ourselves. *Time*, May 28, 2018. pp. 34-39.

3.   Dionne, EJ Jr., Ornstein, NJ, Mann, TE. *One Nation After Trump: A Guide for the Perplexed, the Disillusioned, the Desperate, and the Not-Yet-Deported*. New York. *St. Martin's Press*, 2017, p. 4.

4. Extract from Levitsky, S, Ziblatt, D. *How Democracies Die*. New York. *Crown Publishing Group*, 2018, as quoted by *The Guardian*, January 21, 2018.

5. Berlatsky, N. The Trump effect: New study connects white American intolerance and support for authoritarianism. *NBC News*, May 27, 2018.

6. Gee, E. Estimates of the increase of uninsured by congressional district under the Senate GOP tax bill. *Center For American Progress*, December 5, 2017.

7. Retsinas, J. Cheap insurance: Back to the future. *The Progressive Populist*, June 15, 2018, p. 15.

8. Johnson, CY. Maryland's Obamacare insurers request 30 percent premium hike for 2019. *The Washington Post*, May 7, 2018.

9. Level, NN. Trump's new insurance rules are panned by nearly every healthcare group that submitted formal comments. *Los Angeles Times*, May 30, 2018.

10. Corbett, J. 'Crisis no one is talking about': GOP threatens healthcare of 26 million people. *Common Dreams*, February 2, 2018.

11. Alonzo-Zaldivar, R, Crary, D. Trump remaking federal policy on women's reproductive health. *Association Press*, May 30, 2018.

12. Lawrence, H. As quoted in Ibid # 10.

13. Chittister, J. D (https://www.inspiringquotes.us/author/4564-joan-d-chittister).

14. Itkowitz, D, Somashekhar, S. States prepare to shut down children's health programs if Congress doesn't act. *The Washington Post*, November 23, 2017.

15. Davio, K. Single-payer system is the solution for mental health care, panelists say. *American Journal of Managed Care*, May 7, 2018.

16. Ollove, M. Amid shortage of psychiatric beds, mentally ill face long waits for treatment. *The Pew Charitable Trusts*. Stateline. August 2, 2016.

17. Artiga, S. Disparities in health and health care: Five key questions and answers. Issue Brief. *Kaiser Family Foundation*, August 12, 2016.

18. 2018 Scorecard on State Health System Performance. New York. *The Commonwealth Fund*.

19. Dwyer-Lindgren, L, Bertozi-Villa, A, Stubbs, RW. Trends and patterns of geographic variation in mortality from substance abuse disorders and intentional injuries among U. S. counties, 1980-2014. *JAMA* 319 (10):

1013-1023, 2018.

20.   McKay, B, Rigdon, R. 'Deaths of despair' take toll across U. S. *Wall Street Journal*, April 11, 2018: A3.

21.   Geiger, HJ. Why we do what we do, speech. Doctors for Global Health, August 2002.

22.   Beal, A. Reframing a national dialogue about health care disparities. *The Commonwealth Fund*, April 27, 2018.

23.   Girod, CS, Hart, SK, Weltz, SA. 2018 Milliman Medical Index. *Milliman Research Report*, May 21, 2018.

24.   Altman, D. The medical bill score. How the public judges health care. *Axios*, October 3, 2017.

25.   Luthra, S. When credit scores become casualties of health care. *Kaiser Health News,* May 9, 2018.

26.   Radley, DC, McCarthy, D, Hayes, SL. 2018 Scorecard on State Health System Performance. New York. *The Commonwealth Fund.*

27.   Osborn, R, Doty, MM, Moulds, D et al. Older Americans were sicker and faced more financial barriers to health care than counterparts in other countries. *Health Affairs*, November 15, 2017.

28.   Rau, J. Why glaring quality gaps among nursing homes are likely to grow if Medicaid is cut. *Kaiser Health News,* September 28, 2017.

29.   Aleccia, J, Bailey, M, de Marco, H. No one is coming. Hospice patients abandoned at death's door. *Kaiser Health News*, October 26, 2017.

30.   Abelson, R. United Health buys large doctors group as lines blur in health care. *New York Times*, December 6, 2017.

31.   Tracer, Z. Forget Amazon. Health companies really want to be UnitedHealth. *Bloomberg News*, December 4, 2017.

32.   de la Merced, MJ, Abelson, R. CVS to buy Aetna for $69 billion in a deal that may reshape the health industry. *New York Times*, December 3, 2017.

33.   Abelson, R. Hospital giants vie for patients in effort to fend off new rivals. *New York Times*, December 18, 2017.

34.   Abelson, R, Sanger-Katz, M, Creswell, J. As an insurer resists paying for 'avoidable' E.R. visits, patients and doctors push back. *New York Times*, May 19, 2018.

35.   Alterman, E. Hungry and invisible. *The Nation*, November 13, 2017.

36.   Rampell, C. Congress takes food from 2 million poor people—and doesn't

even save money. *The Washington Post*, May 17, 2018.

37. Waxman, E. How far do SNAP benefits fall short of covering the cost of a meal? *Urban Institute*, February 22, 2018.

38. Galewitz, P. 4 takeaways from Trump's plan to rescind CHIP funding. *Kaiser Health News*, May 8, 2018.

39. Bernstein, J, Katch, H. Cutting support for economically vulnerable women is no way to celebrate Mother's Day. *The Washington Post*, May 11, 2018.

40. Scism, L. Safety net frays for millions of retirees. *Wall Street Journal*, January 17, 2018: A1.

41. Galewitz, P. Medicaid covers all that? It's the backstop of America's ailing health system. *Kaiser Health News*, September 25, 2017.

42. KHN Morning Briefing. Thousands of nursing home residents face eviction due to Louisiana's cuts to Medicaid funding, May 9, 2018.

43. vanden Heuvel, K. Trump's brutal policies target the most vulnerable Americans, *The Progressive Populist*, June 15, 2018, p. 12.

44. Dewey, C. White America's racial resentment is the real impetus to welfare cuts, study says. *The Washington Post*, May 30, 2018.

CHAPTER 15

TRUMPCARE VS. SINGLE-PAYER MEDICARE FOR ALL

We're going to have insurance for everybody. There was a philosophy in some circles that if you can't pay for it, you don't get it. That's not going to happen with us.

—Donald Trump. Statement to
The Washington Post, January 15, 2017. [1]

The above is one of the thousands of lies Trump has made since his presidential candidacy and inauguration. Earlier chapters have made a mockery of this statement as we now know that the private health insurance industry costs much more every year even as it provides less coverage. It satisfies its CEOs and Wall Street shareholders far more than its enrollees. Tens of millions of Americans do not have insurance as insurers pursue ever-higher profits. The industry is on a death march of which the administration and GOP seem unaware. We now have a polarized gap between Republicans and Democrats over how to proceed in reforming health care, as well as dissension within both parties as to the next steps to take.

This chapter has just two goals: (1) to compare the two basic alternatives to health care reform—continuance of incremental tweaks to TrumpCare, the sabotaged version of ObamaCare, versus fundamental reform through single-payer Medicare for All; and (2) to consider what the public needs and wants.

Two Basic Alternatives

1. *Continuation of TrumpCare*

As long as Trump occupies the White House and the GOP controls Congress, what we have now is what we get, as described in Chapter 3 (pages 55-61), however failed its policies are. Although a Health Policy Consensus Group has been formed by a group of conservative think tanks that is still trying to repeal the ACA, this appears unlikely to pass given the outcomes of previous efforts. [2] However, Attorney General Jeff Sessions, with Trump's support, has recently decided not to defend in court the constitutionality of the ACA itself, which could end up wiping out whatever remains of patient protections. [3]

Costs will increase

Under the current policies of TrumpCare, the crisis in U. S. health care described in the last chapter will continue unabated, with some problems getting progressively worse as corporate stakeholders take whatever revenues they can make on the backs of patients, families and taxpayers. With deregulation the policy of our times, we cannot expect any containment of the costs of insurance and health care, while the rolls of the uninsured increase and the epidemic of underinsurance only gets worse. [4] As Robert Reich comments:

> *Health insurers spend lots of time, effort, and money trying to attract people who have high odds of staying healthy (the young and fit) while doing what they can to fend off those who have high odds of getting sick (the older, infirm, and unfit). As a result we end up with the most bizarre health insurance system imaginable: One ever more carefully designed to avoid sick people.* [5]

Short-term plans with limited coverage increase

Insurers can exclude coverage for pre-existing conditions, and are not obligated to extend coverage beyond one year without medical underwriting. The administration's promotion of short-term plans may appeal to many healthy people, but will restrict coverage for such categories as preventive services, maternity care, mental health care, and prescription drugs. Many purchasers of short-term plans will be sorely disappointed, warns Sabrina Corlette, a research professor at Georgetown University's Health Policy Institute:

> *People should be aware. There's a huge variety of plans out there—from true bottom feeders that are going to take your money and don't provide any protection to legitimate products that are designed to meet a short-term need.* [6]

Paul Spitalnic, Medicare's chief actuary, estimates that 1.4 million people could sign up for short-term plans in the first year. Because those remaining in the ACA's martketplaces will be relatively less healthy, he predicts that premiums will rise further in those markets, increasing federal spending by $1.2 billion in 2019. [7]

Increasing privatization

The administration's promotion of increasing privatization ignores the higher costs, restricted access, lower quality of care, and less accountability which will result. Here are examples of profiteering by privatized Medicare and Medicaid plans with worse care. Sicker patients on Medicare Advantage plans frequently leave their plans as insurers cut access to preferred physicians, hospitals, and necessary drug treatment. Freedom Health, one such insurer in Florida, paid out almost $32 million in a 2017 settlement of allegations that it exaggerated how sick patients were to increase profits while dropping others who were costing them too much. [8]

Congress has just passed a new Chronic Care Act that received bipartisan support and fits within the Trump administration's pressure toward increased privatization. It is intended to provide extra benefits to patients with multiple chronic illnesses, including such additional benefits as home improvements like wheelchair ramps, transportation to doctors' offices, and home delivery of hot meals. Who can argue with that? The problem is that these new benefits will only be offered through Medicare Advantage, privatized Medicare, not through traditional public Medicare. This will end up as a bait and switch strategy that will threaten the survival of Medicare itself. Private insurers, of course, strongly support this new law, while Seema Verma, head of CMS, of course calls this "a big win for patients." [9]

Dr. Don McCanne sees through this plot this way:

This is another blatant effort to privatize Medicare by providing more funds and better benefits through the private plans while depriving the traditional Medicare program from such funding. Once enough Medicare beneficiaries transfer to the private plans, our government stewards can move forward with their plan to devitalize the traditional program, reducing it to a shrunken, underfunded welfare program if not totally shutting it down. . . . By infusing the private plans with ever more cash while depriving the traditional program of adequate funds, they will appear to have proved that competing private plans are superior to the public program, when, in fact, the private plans are being paid significantly more than is the cost of the public program for patients of comparable health status. The claim of lower costs through competition of private Medicare Advantage plans is a fraud. [10]

Privatization of the Veterans Administration is another example of goals and promises of TrumpCare going the wrong way. Under the new program, VA Choice, veterans often have to wait between 51 and 64 days for appointments with private physicians. Because of poor communication through electronic medical records, they may have to wait for months to discuss treatment options after an MRI of the neck and lower back. [11] Yet Trump lies once again in defending the new VA Choice program (even while the White House opposes its funding) by saying that [going outside the VA to a private doctor] "is less expensive for us, it works out much better and it's immediate care. And that's what we're doing." [12]

Prescription drugs with continuing high costs

The costs of prescription drugs exposes the charade of Trump's promises. In a May 2018 speech, Trump vowed to "bring soaring drug prices back to earth by promoting competition among pharmaceutical companies." He further stated:

> *Everyone involved in the broken system—the drugmakers, insurance companies, pharmacy benefit managers and many others—contribute to the problem. Government has also been part of the problem because previous leaders turned a blind eye to this incredible abuse. But under this administration we are putting American patients first.* [13]

But Trump is not putting patients first, for he rejected having the federal government negotiate drug prices (as the VA has done for years in getting discounts down to 58 percent of what we pay) and did not allow importation of lower-cost drugs from abroad.

DHHS Secretary Alex Azar served as former head of Eli Lilly's U. S. division from 2012 to 2017, during which time the price of its insulin drug Humalog more than doubled from $122 per vial to $274 per vial.[14] Not surprisingly, he, like Trump, rejected out of hand the government's role in negotiating drug prices, as most advanced countries have done for many years, in these factually incorrect words:

> *The only way that direct negotiation could possibly save money is by doing something this administration doesn't believe in: denying access to certain medicines for all Medicare beneficiaries through rationing, or setting prices for drugs by government fiat.* [15]

Instead, the administration is proposing consolidation of coverage for all prescription medicines under Medicare's Part D program as a way to lower spending on drugs. This proposal ran quickly into a brick wall with PhRMA, which expressed serious concerns that this would limit patient affordability and access. It turns out that drug companies make much more money from our current system whereby under Medicare Part B, the government pays a drug's average sales price plus 6 percent. [16]

Primary care access limited

Primary care will be further split as the battle between insurers and hospital systems plays out over control of primary care patients. The vacuum in primary care will continue as the rates of burnout among primary health care professionals increase and get worse in the absence of any federal workforce plan. Urgent care and various forms of retail walk-in clinics will further multiply, thereby further fragmenting care that results in worse outcomes of care and higher patient dissatisfaction with this non-system.

State block grants with less health care for many

Allowing states more responsibility for health care, as is contemplated by the GOP through state block grants, will worsen access and outcomes of care, and further increase health disparities. Eligibility for Medicaid is already extremely restrictive in many states, such as Alabama, Kansas, Maine, Mississippi, North Carolina and Wisconsin. In Alabama, for example, one cannot qualify for Medicaid with an annual income more than 18 percent of the federal poverty level (about $312 a month). [17] In Louisiana, only 26 percent of Medicaid enrollees with high blood pressure have adequate control of it, while just 21 percent of women receive post-partum checkups.[18]

2. Single-Payer Medicare for All

In sharp contrast to TrumpCare, single-payer Medicare for All, as represented by H. R. 676 in the House, as soon as it is enacted, will bring:

- Universal access to health care for all Americans from day one, with all providers and hospitals "in network."
- Coverage of all medically necessary care, including inpatient and outpatient services, prescription drugs, reproductive health, mental health, dental, vision, and long-term care.
- Coverage of 100 percent of health care costs without premiums, copays or deductibles.
- Administrative simplification with efficiencies and cost containment through large-scale cost controls, including global budgeting of hospitals and other facilities, negotiated fee schedules, and bulk purchasing of drugs and medical devices.
- Transition over 15 years from a largely for-profit system to a not-for-profit, service-oriented system.
- Pharmaceutical reform, including independent and rigorous evaluation of the efficacy and safety of medications.

- Elimination of the private health insurance industry, with its
  large, increasing administrative overhead and profiteering
  converted to cost savings that enable universal coverage
  through a non-profit financing system.

Benefits to patients

With their new Medicare for All cards assuring coverage under
national health insurance (NHI), patients will just present their
cards when seeking care. The administrative overhead of the new
system will be cut by five-fold. Patients will have full choice of
physicians and other providers, who will be in private practice, not
employees of the government, and who will see a sharp reduction
in their overhead and administrative tasks, allowing more time for
direct patient care. Reimbursement for primary care physicians and
other shortage specialties, such as psychiatry and geriatrics, will be
increased. With stronger primary care, today's fragmented care will
be better coordinated.

Lower costs of national health insurance

A classic study by Gerald Friedman, professor of economics
at the University of Massachusetts, projects the NHI will save
about $592 billion annually by cutting out administrative waste of
private insurers ($476 billion) and reducing pharmaceutical prices
to European levels ($116 billion) through negotiated drug prices and
bulk purchasing. [19]

As a result of these savings, 95 percent of Americans will pay less
than they now do for insurance and health care under a progressive
tax system. Those with annual incomes of $50,000 will pay $1,500 in
taxes, increasing to $6,000 for incomes of $100,000 and $12,000 for
incomes of $200,000 a year. [20] Recall that the average family of four
now pays $28,000 per year for health insurance and care. Federal and
state governments will save money, as will taxpayers, in a simplified

Table 15.1

HOW SINGLE-PAYER NHI WILL IMPROVE QUALITY OF CARE

Access	• Everyone automatically eligible/ensured access; only plan for true universal insurance and access. • Able to control cost globally (w/ fences) so no reliance on access barriers to maintain affordability.
User-Friendly Simple	• A "no depends" system-no complicated rules, exchanges, variations by age, state, income, disease, employment/employer, marital status, etc. • Avoids eligibility determinations, means testing,confusion, enrollment complexities.
Single Standard	• By definition single system with fair rules for all • Generates database to identify disparities and track effectiveness of interventions
Continuity	• No switching for change in employment, divorce, new private insurance plan, restricted networks • Ensured reimbursement permitting provider financial stability.
Choice	• Avoids negative features and restricted networks, choice of provider and hospitals. • Uniform reimbursement and benefits package enables portability and ability to choose
Nursing	• Stable source of funding for hospitals via global budgets • Potentials for national standards, support for nursing education, less frustrations with arbitrary financially-driven anti-nurse cost cutting
Time	• All patients would be covered; ensuring provider is reimbursed for his/her time w/ each. • Greater potential for support of teamwork resulting from continuities of patients, staff, funding
Caring Commitment	• Elimination of greed, profit, corporate controls as the drivers health care system decision making • Restoring ability of professionals to advocate for patients and a better system, rather than current structured antagonisms
Clinical Information Systems	• Role and necessity of national standards, federal leadership in funding IT, demonstrated VA leadership, other countries lead • Design for clinical needs of patients, providers, not insurers, vendors (accountablity w/ unified system) • Ability to collect and aggregate data for quality oversight
Communication	• Better positioned to overcome trade secrets/secrecy inherent in private control • In avoiding financial barriers for patients to seek care, call, lower threshold/barriers for communication.
Continuous Improvement	• Stable public systems, "in business of health" for the long haul thus ROI on quality investment • Noteworthy successes of CQI in public sector (VA,Navy)
Accountability	• Public system by definition public & accountable, especially if democratic decision-making, organized advocacy efforts, vigilant media scrutiny, • Role that Medicare, Medicaid (and hence public insurance data) has played in outcomes evaluation and review of allocation decisions.
Prevention Oriented	• Unlike private plans where prevention does not pay due to frequent patient switches, greater incentives for prevention • Public system can be best integrated with public health at local and national levels

new system that assures ready access to care based on medical need, not ability to pay.

Improved quality of care

Table 15.1 (on previous page) lists many ways by which NHI will improve quality of care for both individuals and population groups, as conceptualized by Dr. Gordon Schiff, associate professor of medicine at Harvard Medical School. [21]

There are two bills in Congress now for universal coverage through Medicare for All. The House version, H. R. 676, with Rep. Keith Ellison as the lead sponsor and more than one-half of House Democrats as co-sponsors, and the Senate version, S. 1804, introduced last year by Sen. Bernie Sanders with 17 co-sponsors. Table 15.2 compares these two bills.

What Does the Public Need and Want?

The needs for Americans in health care come clear in the crisis described in the last chapter. The goals for reform should place the best interests of patients, their families, and the public at the center of reform efforts, not the interests of corporate stakeholders in the medical-industrial complex. Our goals should be to develop a new system that provides universal access to necessary health care that is affordable, comprehensive, efficient, equitable, and sustainable. Most other advanced countries around the world have done that long ago. Why can't we join them now?

After the GOP's final Senate bill collapsed in July 2017, the Editorial Board of *The Washington Post* observed:

> *Congressional Republicans' misguided effort to reshape the U. S. health care system . . . had the virtue of clarifying where the country now stands nearly two decades into the 21st century: Americans want universal health care coverage, including for*

the poor and sick, and they expect the government to ensure that it is provided. Republicans and Democrats can argue about how to meet this end—but if they are wise they will no longer dispute the goal. [22]

Dr. David Ansell, author of the 2017 book, *The Death Gap: How Inequality Kills*, sums up the situation this way:

> *The right to health care in America is not an issue of the left or the right. It's a matter of right and wrong.* [23]

Natalie Shure, researcher and writer whose work focuses on history, health, and politics, makes a compelling feminist case for single-payer NHI, but also sees it as a non-gender issue. In her words:

> *The dynamics that make the American health care system so hostile to women remain largely unscathed after the ACA: the pervasive commodification of healthcare and dependent care in the United States, coupled with employment-based gatekeeping, engineers an impossible bind for women: they face more challenges accessing the health care system and pay more for their care when they do, out of lower incomes that are further squeezed by child and elder care costs.*

> *By removing power over health care from employers and spouses, and replacing unequal tiers with one unified insurance pool, we could fund our health care system with progressive taxes. That way, we could guarantee everyone the care they need, and make it free at the point of service. Ability to pay, pre-existing conditions, employment status, and gender would cease to be barriers.* [24]

TABLE 15.2
COMPARISON OF HOUSE AND SENATE MEDICARE FOR ALL BILLS

	HOUSE: HR 676	SENATE: S 1804
Universality	All residents as defined by Sec. HHS, presumed eligible when present for care.	All residents as defined by Sec. HHS when fully implemented (4 years after passage), doesn't presume inclusion.
Coverage	"All medically necessary care" Includes primary care and prevention, nutrition, inpatient, outpatient, emergency, pharmaceuticals, medical equipment, long term care, palliative care, mental health, dental, substance abuse treatment, chiropractic, vision, hearing, podiatry. Prioritizes in-home and community-based care.	Covered services "if medically necessary or appropriate" Includes primary care and prevention, inpatient, outpatient, emergency, pharmaceutical (specifies biologicals), medical devices, mental, substance abuse treatment, labs and diagnostics, comprehensive reproductive care, dental, hearing and vision, short-term rehabilitative care.
Long Term Care	Covered.	Remains in Medicaid, administered by the states.
Adding benefits	No specific mechanism, perhaps under recommendation of the National Board of Universal Quality and Access (NBUQA).	Specifies adding appropriate complementary and integrative practices and overcoming barriers to care. Includes appeals process.
Cost sharing	None.	Co-pays on pharmaceuticals with exceptions, cap of $200/year.
Choice of provider	Choice of all participating providers in U.S. and territories.	Choice of all participating providers in U.S. and territories.
Providers	All who meet standards and are public or nonprofit (bans investor-owned facilities and phases them out over 15 years). All facilities must meet standards for staffing and quality.	All who meet standards. Includes investor-owned facilities. All facilities must meet standards of staffing, competence, quality and satisfaction.
Opt - out	Not specified.	Providers may opt out but must do so completely. Patients may purchase covered services from providers that opt out and still be covered for other services in the system.
Duplication	No private insurance or HMO that operates as a private insurance can duplicate coverage.	No private insurance can duplicate coverage.
Supplemental insurance	Enrollees can purchase supplemental insurance.	Enrollees can purchase supplemental insurance.
Payment for services	Fees negotiated with NBUQA with input from state physician review boards, determined regionally, paid within 30 days. Alternatives are salary for an institution and capitated payment.	Fees set by Sec. HHS with input, based on current Medicare structure. Includes innovation within MACRA.

Administration	Sec. HHS appoints a general director who appoints long term care and mental health care directors and director for Office of Quality Control, who consults with regional and state directors. State physician review boards. NBUQA is a 15-member stakeholder board appointed by President with Senate approval.	Sec. HHS oversees the entire system and may consult with other agencies and stakeholders. Sec. HHS appoints regional and state directors, regional directors to represent Native American and Native Alaskan tribes, Omsbudsman.
Operating and capital expense budgets	Global operating budgets for each facility and separate capital expense budgets, cannot co-mingle.	No global operating budgets. Facilities can co-mingle operating and capital budgets. No mechanisms to control budgets.
Health Professional Education	Included in general budget.	Included in general budget. Establish Office of Primary Care in AHRQ to expand access to primary care.
Prices for goods	Pharmaceutical, medical supplies and equipment negotiated annually, formulary.	Pharmaceutical, medical supplies and equipment negotiated annually, formulary.
Transition for workers	Displaced workers have first priority to be hired into new system, 2 years salary and training support.	Temporary worker assistance for up to 5 years, capped at 1% of total budget.
Health records	Confidential electronic records, patients can withhold electronic sharing.	Not specified.
Health planning	Annual review. Recommendations come from the states and Office of Quality Control.	Annual review. Audit every 5 years. Input comes from state directors and others as requested.
Veterans/Indian Health	VA/ IHS separate at first. Integrate IHS after 5 years. Evaluate inclusion of VA after 10 years.	VA/IHS remain separate.
Quality control	NBUQA (diverse membership), long term and mental health directors, director of Office of Quality control, regional and state directors all monitor, report, make suggestions and implement.	Overseen by Sec. HHS with input, mechanism for enrollees to appeal and to protect whistleblowers who report violations.
Funding	Medicare Trust Fund includes current public health dollars, various taxes on wealthy, payroll tax. Additional annual sums as necessary.	Medicare Trust Fund includes current public health dollars, otherwise not defined. Reserve fund for emergencies such as epidemics and natural disasters.
Fraud and abuse	Not defined.	As per the Social Security Act.
Start of system	On January 1 of the first year that is more than a year after passage of the Act.	Transition phase begins on January 1 of the first year after passage of the act and lasts 4 years (see chart).
Transition	None. Everyone is in the system when it begins.	Multi-payer system over first 4 years that phases people into a universal single payer system when complete.

Concluding comment

In order to pursue urgently needed health care reform, we must first acknowledge the failure of past policies, including dependence on markets that serve themselves instead of the common good, bailouts of the private health insurance industry, deregulation that serves corporate profiteering over the public interest, cost-sharing at the point of care that just sets up financial barriers to needed care, and experiments in payment of physicians that create incentives to game the system and avoid sicker patients.

The political party that enacts universal coverage could govern for many years in this country. David Leonhardt, in a 2017 plea to Republican conservatives, made these points:

The lack of universal health coverage in a wealthy democracy is a severe, unjustifiable, and unnecessary human wrong. As Americans lift this worry from their fellow citizens, they'll discover that they have addressed some other important problems too. They'll find that they have removed one of the most important barriers to entrepreneurship, because people with bright ideas will fear less to quit their jobs through which they get their health care. They'll find they have improved the troubled lives of the white working class succumbing at earlier ages from preventable deaths of despair. They'll find that they have equalized the life chances of different races. They'll find that they have discouraged workplace discrimination against women, older Americans, the disabled, and other employees with higher expected health-care costs. They'll find that their people become less alienated from a country that has become at last one of the least attractive manifestations of American exceptionalism—and joined the rest of the civilized world in ameliorating and alleviating our common human vulnerability to illness and pain. [25]

References:

1. Costa, R, Goldstein, Trump vows 'insurance for everybody' in Obamacare replacement plan. *The Washington Post*, January 15, 2017.

2. Armour, S, Hughes, S. GOP in new push to repeal ACA. *Wall Street Journal*, May 26-27, 2018: A4.

3. Goldstein, A. Trump administration won't defend ACA in case brought by GOP states. *The Washington Post*, June 7, 2018.

4. Editorial Board. *The Washington Post*. Health care is still a mess. Republicans are making it worse, June 4, 2018.

5. Reich, R. Aetna shows why we need single-payer. *Common Dreams*, August 16, 2017.

6. Corlette, S, as quoted by Appleby, J. Desperate for coverage: Are short-term plans better than none at all? *Kaiser Health News*, December 1, 2017.

7. Pear, R. Medicare's own actuary confirms the deleterious consequences of short-term health plans. *New York Times*, May 15, 2018.

8. Schulte, F. As seniors get sicker, they're more likely to drop Medicare Advantage plans. *Kaiser Health News*, July 6, 2017.

9. Pear, R. Medicare allows more benefits for chronically ill, aiming to improve care for millions. *New York Times*, June 25, 2018.

10. McCanne, D. Quote of the Day, June 25, 2018.

11. Yen, H. AP NewsBreak: Long waits under VA's private health program. *Associated Press*, June 4, 2018.

12. Yen, H. AP fact check: Trump's overhaul of vets care is no quick fix. *Associated Press*, June 7, 2018.

13. Pear, R. Trump promises lower drug prices, but drops populist solutions. *New York Times*, May 11, 2018.

14. King, R. DHHS nominee Alex Azar takes heat for rising insulin prices. *Washington Examiner*, November 29, 2017.

15. Pear, R. Trump administration defends plan to lower prescription drug prices. *New York Times*, May 14, 2018.

16. Cunningham, PW. There's a fight brewing between the Trump administration and drugmakers. *The Washington Post*, May 17, 2018.

17. Cunningham, PW. Here are three big ways the Trump administration could put its mark on Medicaid. *The Washington Post*, May 16, 2018.

18. Cunningham, PW. Trump administration rolls out a beauty pageant for Medicaid. *The Washington Post*, June 5, 2018.

19. Friedman, G. Funding H. R. 676: The Expanded and Improved Medicare for All Act. How we can afford a national single-payer health plan. Chicago, Ill. *Physicians for a National Health Program*, July 31, 2013.

20. Woolhandler, S, Himmelstein, DU. Single-payer reform: The only way to fulfill the President's pledge of more coverage, better benefits, and lower costs. *Annals of Internal Medicine online*, February 21, 2017.

21. Dr. Gordon Schiff, personal communication, 2016.

22. Editorial Board, *The Washington Post*, July 28, 2017.

23. Ansell, D. I watched my patients die of poverty for 40 years. It's time for single payer. *The Washington Post*, September 13, 2017.

24. Shure, N. The feminist case for single payer. *Jacobin Magazine*, December 8, 2017.

25. Leonhardt, D. Republicans for single-payer health care. *New York Times*, March 28, 2017.

CHAPTER 16

WINNERS AND LOSERS UNDER TRUMPCARE VS. SINGLE-PAYER MEDICARE FOR ALL

The federal government should not play a huge role in healthcare regulation. The only way the government should be involved, they have to make sure those companies are financially strong, so that if they have a catastrophic event or they have a miscalculation, they have plenty of money. Other than that, it's private.

—Donald Trump, as presidential candidate, in talk to *The Hill* [1]

The above quote is typical of so many by Donald Trump in that it reveals so little understanding of the problems and dynamics of our health care system. It fits with his philosophy and that of congressional Republicans favoring deregulation and a limited role of the federal government in health care.

This chapter has just one goal—to compare the winners and losers under TrumpCare vs. single-payer NHI. The former is dedicated to the interests of the few, especially corporate stakeholders and their shareholders pursuing profits over service to patients. The latter is committed to the common good, whether patients, their families, or taxpayers, through assurance by government that all Americans will benefit from an efficient and sustainable service-oriented system.

Table 16.1 outlines who wins and who loses under TrumpCare.

TABLE 16.1

WINNERS AND LOSERS UNDER TRUMPCARE

Winners	Losers
Large corporate mergers	Patients with pre-existing conditions,
Private health insurers	chronic illness, women, mentally ill,
Drug industry	early retirees, elderly.
Corporate CEOs	Newly uninsured and underinsured
Shareholders	Medicaid beneficiaries through cuts
Wall Street	Physicians and other health professionals
Lobbyists	Rural hospitals
	Taxpayers

Winners

In the hands-off, deregulated approach being taken by the Trump administration to health care, corporate interests thrive as they pursue their self-interest in a profit-driven business ethos. In most cases, they are able to set their own prices, and they have found many ways to game the system. Financially driven coding systems that physicians must fill out for services rendered, often under pressure of their revenue-oriented employers, are at the center of many of these transactions, especially within enlarging hospital systems. In Chapters 11 and 12 we saw how pervasive profiteering, waste, corruption and even fraud are within the current system.

There is currently a hot battle going on between hospitals and insurers over emergency room care. Costs for E. R. visits across the country doubled between 2009 and 2016 without any increase in the number of patients seen. In reaction, some insurers are refusing to pay for visits that they deem unnecessary, putting some patients at risk and fueling hot disputes between hospitals, physicians and insurers. [2]

Private insurers continue to win under TrumpCare as the administration bends to their cries for help. A recent example is the reversal of Trump's previous policy of suspending risk adjustment payments to insurers, supposedly as a way to reduce the increasing premiums to be charged for coverage of sicker people. [3] Another marker of how well insurers are doing is that profit margins for the six top insurers for the first quarter of 2018 were the highest in ten years while their CEOs took in more than $17 million in 2017 [4]

A recent paper published by *The Economist* describes another, even larger source of price-gouging that goes on under the radar—health care firms making excess profits as corporate middlemen. Economists call them "rent seekers," as clarified by this description by Joseph E. Stiglitz, Nobel laureate in economics and former chief economist at the World Bank:

Our political system has increasingly been working in ways that increase the inequality of outcomes and reduce equality of opportunity. This should not come as a surprise: we have a political system that gives inordinate power to those at the top, and they have used that power not only to limit the extent of redistribution but also to shape the rules on the game in their favor, and to extract from the public what can only be called large "gifts." Economists have a name for these activities: they call them rent seeking, getting income not as a reward to creating wealth but by trapping a larger share of the wealth that would otherwise have been produced without their effort. Those at the top have learned to suck out money from the rest in ways that the rest are hardly aware of—that is their true innovation. [5]

In a blog by *The Economist* named after the late Joseph Schumpeter, a leading political economist of his time, estimated numbers are put on this concept in U. S. health care. Health care firms, as the second largest of the largest rent-seeking industries in the country, make a total of $65 billion a year in excess profits through rent seeking, equivalent to $200 per American per year. In more practical terms, these corporate middlemen range from pharmacy benefit managers to preferred provider organizers, who in turn pay doctors, hospitals and pharmacies, which in turn pay wholesalers, who pay manufacturers of equipment and drugs." [6]

Let's see how this plays out in the dark world of drug prices and costs under the Trump administration. Although Trump has pledged to bring drug prices under control, his behavior is the opposite. He has rejected having Medicare negotiate drug prices and also not approved importation of drugs from other countries, both of which could slash prices by large margins. His proposal for the government to expand coverage for all prescription drugs for Medicare beneficiaries under Medicare Part D would force patients to pay more out-of-pocket costs than they now have, especially for very expensive drugs. [7] The drug industry is delighted with this proposal, and shares of drug stocks rose shortly after Trump made this proposal. [8] No surprise here—the drug industry spent more than $171 million lobbying the government in 2017, according to the Center for Responsive Politics.[9]

Then there's the GOP tax plan (scam) passed in December of 2017, widely opposed by Americans across the political spectrum. Three in four Americans (including 70 percent of Republicans) disapproved of the plan as a giveaway to large corporations. Only one-third of responders to the *CBS News* poll felt that it would benefit the middle class. [10]

Losers

Patients are the biggest losers under TrumpCare, whether by losing the ACA's patient protections, losing access because of unaffordable costs, increasingly restrictive insurance coverage if insured, losing Medicaid through cutbacks, being underinsured, or joining the ranks of the uninsured. Women are disadvantaged by the GOP and Trump administration's attacks on reproductive health care and loss of coverage of maternity care in short-term plans. Early retirees face the high costs of insurance and care before becoming eligible for Medicare, which may well face cuts in future GOP budgets. Mental health care is poorly covered by insurance under TrumpCare as many mentally ill continue to be jailed without treatment.

The recent decision by the Attorney General that the Department of Justice will not defend patient protections under the ACA from suits by 20 attorneys general in red states puts restrictions on insurers' and employers' ability to deny coverage based on pre-existing conditions, as well as the ACA itself, in further jeopardy. If the ACA is unraveled in this way, it could adversely impact some 15 million people in the individual market as well as about 175 million people insured by small and large employers. [11] The twenty conservative states are claiming that the entire law is unconstitutional. While the eventual outcome of these suits is unclear, the resulting uncertainty in the insurance market will likely lead to further premium increases.[12]

Patients living in rural areas are at particularly high risk. More than 80 rural hospitals have closed since 2010, with hundreds more in danger of clusure. Although rural hospitals serve a vital role as the hub of accessible care to residents of large areas, it is difficult for these hospitals to recruit and retain physicians and other health professionals and to remain economically viable due to inadequate reimbursement. [13]

Physicians lose by being buried in time-consuming billing and clerical tasks that reduce their time for care of patients. A 2017 report from the National Academy of Medicine found that more than one-half of U. S. physicians are exhibiting signs of burnout, including a "high degree of emotional exhaustion and a low sense of personal accomplishment." [14] The loss of clinical autonomy of today's physicians and other health professionals is summed up by this conclusion of a 2018 report by PwC's Health Research Institute:

The traditional relationship between patients and their health professionals is being displaced by the medical-industrial concept in which physicians, nurses and other professionals are relegated to the workforce while disruptors take control of the reins. [15]

Table 16.2 shows who wins and who loses under Single Payer Medicare for All.

Table 16.2

Winners and Losers under Single-Payer Medicare for All

Winners	Losers
All Americans	Private health insurers
Physicians, other health professionals	Corporate middlemen
Hospitals	Corporate stakeholders
Employers	Privatized Medicare
Mental health care	Privatized Medicaid
Public health	Displaced workers
Federal and state governments	Lobbyists
Taxpayers	

Winners

Patients of all ages, regardless of their health conditions, will be immediately covered with full access to all necessary care, with full choice of provider and hospital, and with no cost sharing at the point of care. This will be a great advance in a new culture of care, which will be affordable for everyone because of sharing risk across all 320 million of us in a more efficient, not-for-profit financing system. Women will gain by having full access to all reproductive health services, thereby gaining control over their own bodies and family choices without political barriers. The new system will be based on medical need, not ability to pay.

As all Americans gain access to all necessary health care, the quality and outcomes of their care will improve, especially for those population subgroups that had inadequate access under the present system. For example, a recent study by the National Academy of Sciences found worse health outcomes in two population subgroups in the aftermath of the Great Recession of 2008 to 2010. Younger adults had to deal with freezing of labor markets, increasing job insecurity, and decline of real income. Older homeowners, not yet retired, who were invested in the stock market, saw declines in their investments as well as home values. Both groups were hard hit with large increases in their blood pressures and blood glucose levels. [16]

Single-payer national health insurance (NHI) will bring equity across the system, provide solid funding of safety net programs in the country, and eliminate today's health care divide from one state to another. NHI will build on the reliable performance demonstrated by traditional, non-privatized Medicare for more than 50 years.

Physicians and other health professionals will join the winners' circle for NHI with administrative simplification and gaining more time for patient care. They will experience higher practice satisfaction, less burnout, and have more autonomy in clinical decision-making. It will be a welcome change to no longer have to deal with the current enormous bureaucracy over pre-authorizations for care and responding to the many restrictions imposed by different private insurers.

With many millions of patients uninsured or underinsured, the hospital industry today is under fire by market forces that compel hundreds of hospitals to shrink, reinvent themselves, or even close.[17] They and other facilities will welcome stabilization of their annual global budgets under NHI.

Employers are increasingly frustrated and burdened by the rising costs of providing employer-sponsored health insurance to their employees. They are starting to get more involved in managing their employees' care instead of paying insurers more every year to do it. One example of this beginning trend is the formation of an independent company to improve health care for the 750,000 employees of Amazon.com Inc., J P Morgan, Chase & Co., and Berkshire Hathaway Inc. [18] Under NHI, these kinds of efforts will no longer be needed as employers are relieved of their role in providing health insurance. They will gain a healthier workforce at less cost, thereby becoming more competitive in a global economy.

Longstanding gaps in coverage of mental health care will be a thing of the past under NHI, which will also provide the opportunity to better fund public health. As was described in the last chapter, federal and state governments, as well as taxpayers, will get far more value in health care through an equitable system of progressive taxation with elimination of today's waste and profiteering of the private multi-payer financing system.

Critics of single-payer NHI say that it will be too disruptive. History tells us the opposite. When Medicare and Medicaid were enacted in 1965, even in a time of 3x5 cards and other paper records, the change was almost seamless for patients and care began right away. When NHI is enacted, individuals will have immediate care available. Disruption will occur, however, in the private administrative sector, but that is needed to rectify its many problems that have been sold to us under the false banner of "more efficiency in the private sector."

Losers

Private health insurers have had their chance for many decades and have failed the common good. The larger labyrinth of corporate middlemen profiteering throughout the medical-industrial complex likewise fails the public interest. Privatized Medicare and Medicaid have shown themselves to have higher costs with profits than the publicly administered programs. This feeding at the public trough at both federal and state levels is unsustainable and will be stopped.

Corporate stakeholders ranging from pharmaceutical companies to medical device manufacturers will have the opportunity to compete based on the quality and efficacy of their products in one big market through bulk purchasing under single-payer NHI.

Among the losers, it is important to note that the House bill for single-payer NHI (H. R. 676) provides for a 15-year transition period to phase out investor-owned for-profit delivery systems. [19] It also includes $51 billion for retraining the 1.7 million workers displaced by its passage. While this number is large, it is far less than the 60 million Americans who are separated from their jobs each year. However, as economist Gerald Friedman points out:

These include, of course, those with bad jobs doing billing and insurance related work. They include owners and management of insurance companies, drug companies and for-profit hospitals, as well as banks who profit from providing financial services to these companies. And they also include management of not-for-profit hospitals and insurance companies who have been piling up reserves to fund lavish salaries and benefit packages. They also include some unions who maintain their staff with the support of union benefit funds and health programs. Together, the opposition from all these groups is crucial to understanding the failure, thus far, of single-payer health reform. [20]

Concluding Comment

In order to evaluate and come to grips as a society with which of these two alternatives to pursue—TrumpCare or single-payer Medicare for All—we must first answer a fundamental question: who is the health care system for? Is it for patients and families or for corporate interests? If the GOP is to hold to its claimed conservative principles, such as maximizing efficiency and choice, enhancing value, lowering costs, and reining in excess bureaucracy, we should be able to reform U. S. health care in the public interest. That becomes the subject of the next and last chapter.

References

1. Rechtoris, M. Donald Trump quotes on healthcare—'Repeal it, replace it, get something great!' *Becker Hospital Review*, August 16, 2016.
2. Rayasam, R, Demco, P. Insurers spark blowback by reducing emergency room coverage. *Politico*, June 12, 2018.
3. Pear, R. Trump administration, in reversal, will resume risk payments to health insurers. *New York Times*, July 24, 2018.
4. The high cost of healthcare: Patients see greater cost-shifting and reduced coverage in exchange markets 2014-2018. Physicians for Fair Coverage Research by *Avalere*, July 2018.
5. Stiglitz, JE. *The Price of Inequality: How Today's Divided Society Endangers Our Future*. New York. *W. W. Norton & Company*, 2012.
6. Schumpeter. Which firms profit most from America's health care system? *The Economist*, March 5, 2018.
7. Pear, R. Trump plan to lower drug prices could increase costs for some patients. *New York Times*, June 2, 1018.
8. Radovsky, L, Armour, S, Walker, J. Drug industry relieved by price proposal. *Wall Street Journal*, May 12-13, 2018: A1.
9. Reich, R. Trump's drug plan shows he isn't willing to take on Big PhRMA. *The Progressive Populist*, June 15, 2018, p. 13.
10. Corbett, J. Even Republican voters admit widely opposed GOP tax scam is a corporate giveaway. *Common Dreams*, December 7, 2017.
11. Armour, S. Health-law suit touches wider market. *Wall Street Journal*, June 14, 2018.
12. Rovner, J, Appleby, J. Administration challenges ACA's pre-existing conditions protection in court. *Kaiser Health News*, June 8, 2018.
13. Kacik, A. Rethinking rural health care: Rural hospitals look for help to survive. *Modern Healthcare*, June 11, 2018.
14. Clinician well-being is essential for safe, high-quality patient care. *National Academy of Medicine*. Washington, D.C., 2017.
15. *PwC*. Medical cost trend: Behind the numbers, June 2018.
16. PNAS. The Great Recession worsened blood pressure and blood glucose levels in American adults. Seeman, T, Thomas, D, Stein Merkin, S et al. *Proceedings of the National Academy of Sciences*, March 27, 2018.

17. Lauerman, J, Greifeld, K. As U. S. hospital stocks soar, the industry's many ills linger. *Bloomberg News*, March 28, 2017.
18. Humer, C. Fed up with rising costs, big U. S. firms dig into health care. *Reuters*, June 11, 2018.
19. Friedman, G. Funding H. R. 676: The Expanded and Improved Medicare for All Act. How We Can Afford a National Single-Payer Health Plan. *Physicians for a National Health Program*. Chicago, IL, July 31, 2013.
20. Friedman, G. As quoted by Rosenfeld, S. Eleven steps for states to rein in costs while building toward single-payer. *Truthout*, August 11, 2017.

CHAPTER 17

HOW CAN HEALTH CARE BE REFORMED BY 2021?

Of all the forms of inequality, injustice in health care is the most shocking and inhumane. I see no alternative to direct action and creative nonviolence to raise the conscience of the nation.

—Rev. Dr. Martin Luther King, Jr., in a press conference
in Chicago before his speech at the second convention of the
Medical Committee for Human Rights, March 25, 1966. [1]

This above statement by Martin Luther King, Jr. 52 years ago was a wake-up call then, just as it is today, given what we've seen in Chapter 14 about today's crisis in U. S. health care. We need a grassroots backlash to the unfair and cruel market-based system controlled by large corporate stakeholders on the backs of ordinary Americans.

This chapter has three goals: (1) to briefly discuss what we should learn from past failed reform efforts; (2) to describe the battleground over which reform of health care will be fought in Congress and in the states; and (3) to summarize increasing momentum toward Medicare for All, including a time frame as to how this effort could well succeed after the 2020 election cycle.

Repeated Reform Failures due to Misguided Ideology

Before we can proceed to reform U. S. health care, we first need to revisit our assumptions concerning past and current health care policies. We need to learn the lessons discussed in Chapter 1 (see pages 17-23), especially related to the need to change how health care is financed. TrumpCare has depended on failed ideology, perpetuated over many decades, that competitive markets will solve system problems, control prices and costs, and that the private sector is better and more efficient than the public sector.

Chapters 3 to 7 describe TrumpCare under the GOP and Trump administration, including declining access and affordability of care, loss of patient protections, increasing privatization, deregulation of health insurance and care, and shifting responsibility for health care to the states. Chapters 8 to 13 describe the many ways that Trump-Care is failing and how it is not sustainable. In addition to leaving more and more of our population without access to affordable care, and with worse quality and outcomes of care, it is immoral and an increasing drain on the public purse.

What can we learn from the failures of TrumpCare, and likewise from its predecessor, the ACA? Perhaps most important, both programs relied on competitive markets and a multi-payer financing system. We have learned that these markets have wide latitude to set prices and that cost containment is nowhere in sight. We have learned that the private health insurance industry receives $685 billion in government subsidies each year, and that the CBO projects this number to double in another ten years. [2] Insurers have segmented markets to their advantage, and are on a death march that is still under-recognized by legislators. Health care has just become another commodity to be bought and sold within a deregulated marketplace that maximizes revenues to providers at the expense of patients and their families. Under TrumpCare, physicians and other health care professionals are relegated to the status of employed workers and are increasingly burning out.

It is long past time when we should learn from history, especially from the wisdom of leaders in earlier times. Dr. Henry Sigerist,

Director of the History of Medicine at the John Hopkins University, made this key observation as far back as 1944:

Illness is an unpredictable risk for the individual family, but we know fairly accurately how much illness a large group of people will have, how much medical care they will require, and how many days they will have to spend in hospitals. In other words, we cannot budget the cost of illness for the individual family but we can budget it for the nation. The principle must be to spread the risk among as many people as possible . . . The experience of the last 15 years in the United States [since 1931] has, in my opinion, demonstrated that voluntary health insurance does not solve the problem of the nation. It reaches only certain groups and is always at the mercy of economic fluctuations . . . Hence, if we decide to finance medical services through insurance, the insurance system must be compulsory. [3]

Kenneth Arrow, a leading economist at Columbia University, predicted in 1963 that uncertainty would be the root cause of market failure in health care, both for patients and physicians dealing with the unavoidable uncertainties concerning diagnosis, treatment, and prognosis of illness. [4]

Robert Reich brings us right up to date with this challenge:

The real choice in the future is either a hugely expensive for-profit oligopoly with the market power to charge high prices even to healthy people and stop insuring sick people. Or else a government-run single-payer system—such as is in place in almost every other advanced economy—dedicated to lower premiums and better care for everyone. We're going to have to choose eventually. [5]

It is especially interesting to note how conservatives in other advanced countries around the world respond to this challenge based on their moral principles. Donald Light, Ph.D., co-author of the important 1996 book, *Benchmarks for Fairness for Health Care Reform*, observed that conservatives in every other industrialized country have long supported universal access to necessary health care on the basis of four conservative moral principles—anti-free-riding, personal integrity, equal opportunity, and just sharing. In a 2002 paper, he laid out these guidelines for conservatives to stay true to their principles:

1. Everyone is covered, and everyone contributes in proportion to his or her income.
2. Decisions about all matters are open and publicly debated. Accountability for costs, quality and value of providers, suppliers, and administrators is public.
3. Contributions do not discriminate by type of illness or ability to pay.
4. Coverage does not discriminate by type of illness or ability to pay.
5. Coverage responds first to medical need and suffering.
6. Nonfinancial barriers by class, language, education, and geography are to be minimized.
7. Providers are paid fairly and equitably, taking into account their local circumstances.
8. Clinical waste is minimized through public health, self-care, prevention, strong primary care, and identification of unnecessary procedures.
9. Financial waste is minimized through simplified administrative arrangements and strong bargaining for good value.

10. Choice is maximized in a common playing field where 90-95 percent of payments go toward necessary and efficient health services and only 5-10 percent to administration [6]

These moral principles are timeless and should serve as key guideposts for reform of our completely dysfunctional health care system.

The Battleground over Health Care Reform

In addition to tens of millions of patients and families, many corporate stakeholders within the medical-industrial complex are also unhappy under TrumpCare. Big PhRMA, America's Health Insurance Plans (AHIP), hospitals, and health care professionals are all unhappy with the turmoil and continuing threats to their futures. Wall Street is vulnerable to volatility and uncertainty within health care markets. Increasing public dissatisfaction will likely expand public awareness and support for real reform that will stop the leakage from their pocketbooks and give them more choice and real access to actual care.

Meanwhile, the ACA is not dead. It continues to be popular, with almost 12 million people having enrolled in 2018. [7] Four of five of these new signups live in states that Trump carried in the 2016 election. [8] Moreover, three more states have expanded Medicaid since the election, bringing that total to 34, and others are considering doing so, including Idaho, Nebraska, and North Carolina. [9]

Cutbacks in Medicare and Medicaid funding remain a constant threat to both of these programs, together with the Trump administration's continued push to privatize them. The legal case brought by 20 states attorneys general to protect provisions of the ACA remains undecided. [10]

What to do about Medicaid is still a hot issue at both federal and state levels. Medicaid, the nation's largest health program, covers about 75 million Americans, one-half of whom are children. Seema Verma, CMS administrator, sees it as two different programs—"one that serves the most fragile, vulnerable populations in our society . . . the other a program for able-bodied individuals." [11] Hence, the administration's new work requirements for Medicaid beneficiaries, with little regard for the facts that many are disabled, have chronic illness, and often are already working. State governments are facing—with more responsibility for Medicaid and less federal money—the prospect of losing money as they try to implement these new rules. [12]

With the intent to gather more information about how Medicaid is performing across the country, CMS has just released a Medicaid "scorecard" that has been loudly panned by the National Association of Medicaid Directors as inaccurate, incomplete, non-transparent, and less than useful. Sara Rosenbaum, professor of health law and policy at George Washington University, who previously led a congressional advisory board on Medicaid, found the information "too incomplete to be of great value," and further:

> *It's amazing to me that in 2018 this is all we have when trying to understand how the nation's largest insurer performs for its poorest and most vulnerable residents.* [13]

Divisions within the GOP

The GOP in Congress has boxed itself into a corner of its own making. Complicit with the Trump administration's efforts to sabotage the ACA after failed attempts to repeal and replace it without a replacement plan, they are left on the defensive in their ownership of TrumpCare. In the aftermath of CSRs going away, insurers are "silver loading" some of their plans in the ACA's marketplaces and raising premiums. Some insurers have already requested rate increases of more than 30 percent for 2019. [14] These increases will be announced before the midterms, leaving many Americans angry about their decreased choices of affordable health insurance.

With the exit of House Speaker Paul Ryan, the primary force for cuts in Social Security, Medicare and Medicaid, GOP efforts to cut entitlements in 2018 appear dim to none. [15,16] Hollowing out of what safety net is left will likely lead to more voters calling for real reform. Republicans are likely to be on the receiving end of anger from voters who see the 2017 tax bill as a giveaway to corporations and the wealthy. It is also unlikely that the GOP will press forward before the midterms with new attempts to unravel the ACA. Republicans are divided between conservatives who had vowed to eliminate the ACA, and moderates, some in tough election races, who want to preserve its popular protections of those who are sick. [17] Republicans running in competitive districts are already voicing support for guaranteed coverage of pre-existing conditions.[18] A March 2018 *Wall Street Journal/NBC News* poll found that 50 percent of respondents want the Democrats to control Congress, with 40 percent supporting Republican control. [19]

What we can expect of the GOP, however, is a united effort to discredit single-payer Medicare for All through this kind of disingenuous disinformation:

- "Single-payer Medicare for All is socialized medicine."
  Fact: Physicians, other health professionals, hospitals and most other facilities remain in private hands, not owned or employed by the government.

- "Single-payer will lead to rationing of care." *Fact:* Completely the opposite; TrumpCare already severely rations care to the many millions of people who can't afford insurance or care, and for those "insured" who can no longer count on adequate coverage.
- "Costs will skyrocket under single-payer." *Fact:* Single-payer is the *only* approach to health care reform that can control prices and costs of care. Table 17.1 shows annual savings that will accrue after single-payer is enacted. [20]
- "We can't afford single-payer." *Fact:* Not only will single-payer bring universal coverage to all Americans for all necessary health care through these cost savings, 95 percent of Americans can expect to pay less than they do now through a system of progressive taxation. Figure 17.1 shows the change in after-tax household income by income group of taxpayers. Those with incomes less than $250,000 a year pay less, while those with higher incomes pay more. [21]
- "Single-payer will be too disruptive." *Fact:* How can health care be more disruptive than it is now?! Instead, single-payer will immediately start to correct today's system problems, in the same seamless way that the enactment of Medicare and Medicaid happened in the mid-1960s.

Divisions among the Democrats

Like the Republicans, the Democrats are divided between centrists who still defend and take credit for the ACA and the Bernie Sanders-led progressive wing of the party. The division was made clear in the aftermath of the race for the chairmanship of the Democratic National Committee between Thomas Perez and Keith Ellison, which Perez won by a narrow 235 vote margin. [22] Since then, Ellison has become the leading sponsor of H. R. Expanded and Improved Medicare for All in the House, while Perez still resists putting it on the party's platform.

Table 17.1

ANNUAL SAVINGS WITH SINGLE-PAYER REFORM
(In Billions)

Insurance overhead & administration of public programs	220.0
Hospital administration and billing	149.3
Physicians' office administration and billing	75.3
Total administration	503.6
Outpatient prescription drugs	113.2
Total administration plus outpatient prescription drugs	616.8

Source: Woolhandler, S, Himmelstein, DU. Single-payer reform: The only way to fulfill the President's pledge of more coverage, better benefits, and lower costs. *Annals of Internal Medicine online*, February 21, 2017.

The Center for American Progress (CAP), a prominent liberal think tank, has introduced its "Medicare Extra for All" proposal as a potential incremental step toward single-payer. Its vaguely worded proposal would build on Medicare, but has no method for its financing and preserves the private insurance industry, a big part of our current problems. It seems to be an effort to confuse the public, to sound good to the uninformed, and to please their campaign donors.[23] Other centrists argue for bringing back the public option, which RoseAnn DeMoro, president of National Nurses United, correctly labels as "fools gold." [24] She further adds that single-payer should be a litmus test for Democrats with these words:

It's a clarifying issue like none I've ever seen. We're talking about people's lives and health and money. [25]

Figure 17.1

CHANGE IN AFTER-TAX HOUSEHOLD INCOME DUE TO ADOPTION OF PROGRESSIVE FINANCING FOR H.R. 676:
95% of Americans are Better Off Under a Single-Payer System

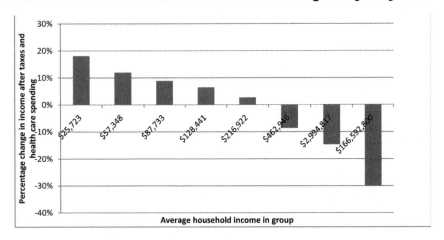

Source: Physicians for a National Health Care Program, April 19, 2017.

Senator Elizabeth Warren (D-MA), author of the 2017 book, *This Fight is Our Fight: The Battle to Save America's Middle Class*, argues that:

Simply blocking the Republican rollback of the Affordable Care Act, also called Obamacare, is not enough to distinguish Democrats from their GOP counterparts in the minds of voters. President Obama tried to move us forward with health care coverage by using a conservative model that came from one of the conservative think tanks that had been advanced by a Republican governor in Massachusetts. Now it's time for the next step. And the next step is single-payer. [26]

Harry Snyder, a consumer advocate and lecturer at the University of California, Berkeley School of Public Health, and Courtney Hutchison, a public health policy advocate, raise and answer this important question:

> *If the threat of TrumpCare breathes new life into single-payer health care, can this lead to real policy change? Not without some serious changes within the Democratic Party . . . [It] has forgotten what it means to lead, to inspire Americans with policies that will work in the long run. Instead, the party is content with a milquetoast incrementalism that counts success in dollars raised and fellow Democrats elected. And it is costing them. It lost them the 2016 election.* [27]

Opposition to Single-Payer Medicare for All from corporate stakeholders

There can be no question that powerful corporate interests across the entire medical-industrial complex want to maintain their very profitable control over U. S health care. Combine that with the myths and memes they will disseminate about single-payer Medicare for All, together with corporate ownership of most of the media, Citizens United, and their track record over the years of countering real health care reform, the odds for progressive reform of health care are indeed daunting. We already know that Democrats not backing Medicare for All get twice as much in campaign donations as co-sponsors of that bill. [28]

As Benjamin Page and Martin Giles say in their important 2017 book, *Democracy in America? What Has Gone Wrong and What Can We Do About It:*

Entrenched interests that benefit from the current system will not relinquish their advantages without a fight. For significant progress to occur, three conditions must be met. First, there must be widespread agreement that we have serious problems—that our society and economy are failing millions of citizens. Second, those failures must be understood, at least in part, as failures of government to respond to the wants and needs of ordinary Americans. And third, enough people must care enough about these problems to devote a lot of time and energy to bring about change. . . . When enough Americans demand change, major moves toward more democracy can be achieved. [29]

This kind of consensus and possible bipartisanship seems unlikely in the present political climate considering how the Senate under McConnell crafted his intent to repeal the ACA—by appointing a secret committee of 13 Republican men to write the bill in total secrecy. As Dionne, Ornstein and Mann have noted in their 2017 book, *One Nation After Trump: A Guide for the Perplexed, the Desperate, and the Not-Yet-Deported*:

That the Senate in the Trump years would set out to upend the American health care system largely in secret was a dramatic and genuinely shocking example of how the decay of norms is not an abstract problem. It threatens the most basic commitments of our democracy. [30]

Increasing Momentum for Medicare for All

According to the latest polls in June 2018 by the *Wall Street Journal/NBC News,* health care is the #1 issue of voters across the political spectrum, even above the economy. [31] Other polls since the start of the Trump presidency have documented increasing support for single-payer Medicare for All. The Pew Research Center found in January 2017 that 60 percent of Americans say the government should be responsible for ensuring health care coverage for all Americans, compared to 51 percent the previous year. [32] A March 2018 poll by the Commonwealth Fund found that 92 percent of adults under age 65 think that all Americans should have the right to affordable health care. [33] A Reuters/Ipsos poll in June and July of 2018 found that 70 percent of American adults support Medicare for All, including 52 percent of Republicans. [34]

Medicare for All has become a leading issue in the Democrat party. A tracking poll by the Kaiser Family Foundation in mid-July 2018 found that three-fourths of respondents say that a single-payer plan for national health insurance should be considered or is very important or the single most important factor in the upcoming midterm elections. [35] A new Medicare for All Caucus has recently been launched by 62 House Democrats. [36]

In order to retake the House in the 2018 midterms, the Democrats need to take 23 seats. In the Senate, they need to hold their present seats and take 2 more to gain control. [37] The odds of a major turnover in Congress in the midterms appears more likely every day.

At the state level, the GOP controls state legislatures in 32 states, but there are many promising developments favoring Democrats as the midterms approach. There are 36 governorships up for grabs this year, together with a large number of down-ballot state offices, such as the all-important state attorney general seats. Eleven Democrats are running for these open governors' seats on a platform of single-payer Medicare for All, including California, Colorado, Florida, Iowa, Maryland, Massachusetts, Michigan, Minnesota, New York, Ohio, and Vermont.[38] As John Nichols, National Affairs correspondent for *The Nation*, predicts:

Riding a 'Blue Wave' into control of statehouses across the country, making red states blue, blue states bluer, and implementing a progressive agenda is not a pipedream; it's the exact inverse of what happened in 2010. [39]

Many progressive organizations are playing a major role in expanding the movement for single-payer health care, including Our Revolution, (which grew out of the Sanders' campaign and has more than 500 chapters in 47 states), Indivisible, Justice Democrats, the Sanders Institute, MoveOn, Public Citizen, Physicians for a National Health Program, Healthcare-NOW!, the American Public Health Association, National Nurses United, and Students for a National Health Program.

Single-payer Medicare for All should be a win-win issue for candidates across much of the country in the 2018 midterms. In response to the Trump administration's attacks on health care at both national and state levels, we have seen dozens of explosive Republican town-hall meetings, dominated by health care and seen by the nation on You Tube. Republican legislators soon began to avoid them because of the anger of the crowds demanding universal health care. [40]

Concluding comment

The battle over health care reform in this country is a litmus test of our democracy. These three closing quotes bring a sense of realism, challenge, and hope as we Americans move forward to resolve the unparalleled problems of U. S. health care.

As Dionne, Ornstein and Mann point out in their 2017 book, *One Nation After Trump: A Guide for the Perplexed, the Disillusioned, the Desperate, and the Not-Yet-Deported*:

*Trumpism represents something far more important than the scheming of one man. To see clearly where Trumpism comes from is to understand that this worldview did **not** just suddenly sweep the country, does **not** command vast support among the American people, and does **not** represent an irresistible wave of the future. But for Trump and Trumpism to be defeated, Americans must understand the nature of the threat that he poses, the shortcomings in our society that he exploited, and the dangers of his overt and covert appeals to racism and xenophobia. They must also embrace public engagement—from demonstrating and attending town meetings to organizing a precinct, registering voters, working on campaigns, running for office, and, of course, voting itself. Saving our democracy requires citizens to devote themselves to the messy, sometimes frustrating, but ultimately gratifying work of self-government.* [41]

Richard Painter, long-time Republican, professor of law at the University of Minnesota, and former ethics lawyer in the George W. Bush administration, has recently decided to switch parties and run as a Democrat for the Senate from Minnesota. He is a supporter of single-payer Medicare for All. Here is what he has to say about the state of play in the upcoming elections:

I don't see Republicans on the ballot for federal office, this year, in any state, who should get support. They have all fallen in line behind President Trump. I think it's critical to our democracy. This isn't about being a Democrat; I'm an American before party. I've been a pain in the rear for the Republican Party, and if I were to continue to be involved in the Democratic Party, I will continue to be a pain in the rear on campaign finance, health care, the environment. I'm not interested in party loyalty issues. I'm interested in policy, in issues, and the right thing to do. [42]

Whether or not we can reform health care in America will test our democracy to the core. David Frum, senior editor at *The Atlantic* and author of the 2018 book, *Trumpocracy: The Corruption of the American Republic,* observes:

The way that liberty must be defended is not with amateur firearms, but with an unwearying insistence on the honesty, integrity, and professionalism of American institutions and those that lead them. We are living through the most dangerous challenge to the free government of the United States than anyone alive has encountered. What happens next is up to you. Don't be afraid. The moment of danger can also be your finest hour as a citizen and an American. [43]

References

1. Galarneau, C. Getting King's words right. *Journal of Health Care for the Poor and Underserved. Johns Hopkins Press*, February 2018.
2. Ockerman, E. It costs $685 billion a year to subsidize U. S. health insurance. *Bloomberg News*, May 23, 2018.
3. Sigerist, HE. Medical care for all the people. *Canadian Journal of Public Health* 35 (7): 258, 1944.
4. Arrow, K. Uncertainty and the welfare economics of medical care. *American Economic Review* 53: 941-973, 1963.
5. Reich, R. Why a single-payer healthcare system is inevitable. *Common Dreams*, August 22, 2016.

6.   Light, D W. A conservative call for universal access to health care. *Penn Bioethics* 9 (4): 4-6, 2002.

7.   Goldstein, A. Nearly 12 million people enrolled in 2018 health coverage under the ACA. *The Washington Post*, April 3, 2017.

8.   *Associated Press*. More than 4 in 5 enrolled in 'Obamacare' are in Trump states. December 22, 2017.

9.   Armour, S. GOP states warm to Medicaid expansion. *Wall Street Journal*, June 15, 2018.

10. Pear, R. Justice Dept. says crucial provisions of Obamacare are unconstitutional. *New York Times*, June 7, 2018.

11. Cunningham, PW. Here are three big ways the Trump administration could put its mark on Medicaid. *The Washington Post*, May 16, 2018.

12. Meyer, H. States face big costs, coverage losses from Medicaid work requirements. *Modern Healthcare*, May 23, 2018.

13. Galewitz, P. Verma unveils state Medicaid scorecard but refuses to judge efforts. *Kaiser Health News*, June 5, 2018.

14. Pear, R. Alex Azar, health secretary, denies sabotaging insurance markets. *New York Times*, June 6, 2018.

15. Radnovsky, L, Timiraos, N. Ryan exit dents odds of entitlement cuts. *Wall Street Journal*, April 13, 2018: A5.

16. Cancryn, A, Feris, S. Republicans give up on Medicare overhaul. *Politico*, June 17, 2018.

17. Goodnough, A, Pear, R, Savage, C. Trump's new plan to dismantle Obamacare comes with political risks. *New York Times*, June 8, 2018.

18. Armour, S, Peterson, K. Focus on health care jolts GOP ahead of midterms. *Wall Street Journal*, June 9-10, 2018: A3.

19. Hook, J. Democrats gain voter favor, as does Trump. *Wall Street Journal*, March 19, 2018: A4.

20. Woolhandler, S, Himmelstein, DU. Single-payer reform: The only way to fulfill the President's pledge of more coverage, better benefits, and lower costs. *Annals of Internal Medicine online*, February 21, 2017.

21. Financing National Improved Medicare for All in the United States. *Physicians for a National Health Program*, Chicago, IL, April 2017.

22. Gallagher, T. The Democratic party left after the Ellison DNC campaign: Unite or fight? *Common Dreams*, March 22, 2017.

23. Cohn, J. The liberal establishment suddenly sounds very ambitious on health care. *The Progressive Populist*, April 1, 2018.

24. Johnson, J. Message to Democrats: Get on board with Medicare for All or go home. *Common Dreams*, June 21, 2017.

25. DeMoro, RA. 'Make your stand': Medicare for All supporters ready to hold Dems to account. *Common Dreams*, August 8, 2017.

26. Warren, E. Speaking to the *Wall Street Journal*. Urging Democrats to go bold, Warren says 'The next step is single-payer. *Common Dreams*, June 26, 2017.

27. Snyder, H, Hutchison, C. The real hurdle to single-payer health care? Scared Democrats. *Sacramento Bee*, July 5, 2017.

28. Conley, J. Dems not backing Medicare for All get twice as much industry cash as co-sponsors. *Common Dreams*, September 14, 2017.

29. Page, BI, Gilens, M. *Democracy in America: What Has Gone Wrong and What We Can Do About It.* Chicago. *University of Chicago Press*, 2017, pp 264-265, 269.

30. Dionne, EJ Jr., Ornstein, NJ, Mann, TE. *One Nation After Trump: A Guide for the Perplexed, the Desperate, and the Not-Yet-Deported.* New York. *St. Martin's Press*, 2017, pp. 79-80.

31. Hellmann, J. Poll: Health care a top issue for voters ahead of midterms. *The Hill*, June 7, 2018.

32. Bialik, K. More Americans say government should ensure health care coverage. *Pew Research Center*, January 13, 2017.

33. Collins, SR, Gunja, MZ, Doty, MM et al. Americans' views on health insurance at the end of a turbulent year. *The Commonwealth Fund*, March 1, 2018.

34. Poll. June and July 2018. *Reuters/Ipsos*.

35. McCanne, D. Taking health care reform to the election booth. Quote of the Day, July 25, 2018.

36. Launch of Medicare for All Caucus met with applause as 62 House Democrats demand healthcare for every American 'from the day they were born.' *Common Dreams*, July 19, 2018.

37. Everett, B, Arkin, J. 2018 elections: Shrinking map boosts Democrats in battle for the Senate. *Politico*, June 15, 2018.

38. Corcoran, M. Single-payer health care takes center stage in gubernatorial races. *Truthout*, March 29, 2018.

39. Nichols, J. Taking it to the states: The coming blue wave offers fifty opportunities for progressive change. *The Progressive*, 17-22, June/July 2018.

40. Ellis, BG. Medicare for All: A win-win issue for candidates in the 2018 midterms. *Truthout*, October 26, 2017.

41. Ibid #30, p.7

42. Painter, R. as quoted by Perry, DM. 'I've been a pain in the rear for the Republican Party': A conversation with Richard Painter. *Pacific Standard*, May 17, 2018.

43. Frum, D. *Trumpocracy: The Corruption of the American Republic.* New York. *HarperCollins*, 2018, p. 235.

Index

A

E

H

I

Issa, Rep. Darrell, bill to protect political spending, 33

J

JAMA Internal Medicine, medical device findings, 111
Johnson, Lyndon, signing Social Security Amendments
Johnson & Johnson ASR hip replacement, 111
Jost, Timothy, Washington and Lee School of Law, insight on Trump's agenda for
        healthcare, 65

K

Kaiser Family Foundation
        analysis of care by race/ethnicity, 212 (Fig. 14.1)
        finding that half of respondents think ACA's marketplaces are falling apart, 265
        finding that three-fourths of respondents think a single-paper plan is important in
                midterm elections, 265
        "medical bill score," 214
        re responsibility for ACA repeal, 53, 54
        short-term policies study in 45 states, 194
        state cost sharing, conclusions, 75
Kaiser Health News, report on drug industry pensions and stock, 34
Kennedy, Ted, single-payer plan, 9
King, Rev. Dr. Martin Luther, 253 (quote re injustice in health care)
Klobuchar, Amy, nursing home concerns, 112 (quote)
Knoer, Scott, 37 (quote as pharmacy officer)
Krugman, Paul, 49 (quote re Trump desire for ACA failure)

L

laboratory tests
        BRCA gene test for cancer, 113
        KIF6 gene test for heart disease, 113
        Wild West of medicine, 113
Laszewski, Robert, industry consultant, 101
Lawrence, Dr. Hal, CEO of American College of Obstetricians and Gynecologists,
        210 (quote)
Leggitt, Larry, 183–184
Legistorm, research company, 34
Leonhardt, David, 1–2, 238–239 (quotes)
Levitsky, *How Democracies Die*, 207 (quote)
Life Care Centers of America Inc., 112
Light, Donald, co-author of *Benchmarks for Fairness for Health Care Reform*, guidelines
        for conservatives, 256–257
Lighty, Michael, California Nurses Association, 69–70 (quote)
lobbying, 18, 30, 31 (Fig. 2.2), 33. *See also* PhRMA
        in administration, 183, 184

N

public health crises: maternal deaths and drug epidemic, 185
Puerto Rico as Medicaid-underfunded, 72–73
Purdue Pharma, OcyContin approval, 186
PwC's Health Research Institute, 246 (quote)

Q

quality of care, failure, 168
    Centers for Disease Control and Prevention, deaths from lack of health insurance, 168
    ECRI Institute finding on patient safety, 168
    inadequate, 214–215
    medical errors and deaths, 168

R

race/ethnicity
    lack of access to care, 212
    racial anxiety, 220
Rampell, Catherine, 51 (quote re Trump against protections)
Rannazzisi, Joe, DEA, 193, 194
Redford, Robert, Board Member of NRDC, 197–198 (quote)
regulation. *See* deregulation of health care
Reich, Robert B., 120, 203, 226, 255–256 (quotes)
Relman, Dr. Arnold, 15–16 (quote re coining term "medical-industrial complex")
Republicans/Republican Congress
    ACA sabotage, 54, 121
    commitment and failure to repeal and replace ACA, 1, 7, 9, 10, 22, 29, 49–50, 234–235
    deregulation favor, 241
    divisions within, 10
    "entitlement funding" position by Gingrich, 1, 70, 80
    House Bill NHI (H.R. 676), 249–250, 262 (Fig. 17.1)
    privatization of Medicare after 1994, 80
    radicalization, 207 (quote by Dionne, Ornstein and Mann)
    tax cut bill, as lie, 2, 196–197
    voter anger at 2017 tax bill, 259
    White Sulphur Springs, West Virginia, retreat, 10
risk pools
    individual mandate repeal, 55
    large, 20
    sharing, 20
    short-term plans, 195
Roosevelt, President Franklin Delano
    backing off NHI, 8
    quote from his reelection speech. 29

T

About the Author

John Geyman, M.D. is professor emeritus of family medicine at the University of Washington School of Medicine in Seattle, where he served as Chairman of the Department of Family Medicine from 1976 to 1990. As a family physician with over 21 years in academic medicine, he also practiced in rural communities for 13 years. He was the founding editor of *The Journal of Family Practice* (1973 to 1990) and the editor of *The Journal of the American Board of* 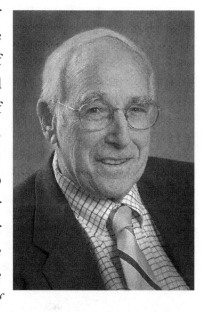 *Family Medicine* from 1990 to 2003. Since 1990 he has been involved with research and writing on health policy and health care reform.

His most recent book was *Crisis in U.S. Health Care: Corporate Power vs. the Common Good* (2017) Earlier books include *The Human Face of ObamaCare: Promises vs. Reality and What Comes Next* (2016), *How Obamacare Is Unsustainable: Why We Need a Single-Payer Solution For All Americans* (2015), *Health Care Wars: How Market Ideology and Corporate Power Are Killing Americans* (2012), *Souls On a Walk: An Enduring Love Story Unbroken by Alzheimer's* (2012), *Breaking Point: How the Primary Care Crisis Threatens the Lives of Americans* (2011), *Hijacked: The Road to Single Payer in the Aftermath of Stolen Health Care Reform (2010),*

The Cancer Generation: Baby Boomers Facing a Perfect Storm (2009), *Do Not Resuscitate: Why the Health Insurance Industry Is Dying (2008), The Corrosion of Medicine: Can the Profession Reclaim Its Moral Legacy* (2008), *Shredding the Social Contract: The Privatization of Medicare* (2006), *Falling Through the Safety Net: Americans Without Health Insurance (2005), The Corporate Transformation of Health Care: Can the Public Interest Still Be Served? (2004),* and *Health Care in America: Can Our Ailing System Be Healed?* (2002).

John has also published two pamphlets following the approach of Thomas Paine in 1775-1776: *Common Sense About Health Care Reform in America* (2017), and *Common Sense: U.S. Health Care at a Crossroads in the 2018 Congress.*

He also served as the president of Physicians for a National Health Program from 2005 to 2007, and is a member of the National Academy of Medicine.

99141473R00188

Made in the USA
Lexington, KY
13 September 2018